Counselling Skills for Nurses

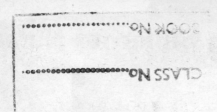

Counselling Skills for Nurses

THIRD EDITION

VERENA TSCHUDIN
BSc (Hons), RGN, RM, Dip. Counselling Skills

Baillière Tindall
London Philadelphia Toronto Sydney Tokyo

Baillière Tindall   24–28 Oval Road
W.B. Saunders   London NW1 7DX, England

The Curtis Center
Independence Square West
Philadelphia, PA 19106–3399, USA

55 Horner Avenue
Toronto, Ontario M8Z 4X6, Canada

Harcourt Brace Jovanovich Group
(Australia) Pty Ltd
30–52 Smidmore Street
Marrickville, NSW 2204, Australia

Harcourt Brace Jovanovich Japan Inc.
Ichibancho Central Building,
22–1 Ichibancho
Chiyoda-ku, Tokyo 102, Japan

First published 1982
Second edition 1987
Reprinted 1988

Typeset by Photo·graphics, Honiton, Devon
Printed in Great Britain by Mackays of Chatham PLC, Chatham, Kent.

British Library Cataloguing in Publication Data

Tschudin, Verena
  Counselling skills for nurses.—3rd edn.
  1. Nursing—Great Britain   2. Counselling
  —Great Britain
  I. Title
  362.1'04256   RT42

ISBN 0–7020–1517–2

Contents

Preface

When *Counselling Skills for Nurses* was first commissioned it was a leap of faith on the part of the publishers. Now, ten years later, books on the subject abound. Titles are becoming ever more daring. And there is room for more.

It seems that as our society is becoming more materialistic, so the human side of it has to be balanced, learned afresh, even discovered. This is exciting. Aspects are uncovered which perhaps are as old as humankind, but they need to be expressed in today's language and idiom. We cannot simply live on the experience of generations ago; to have meaning each person needs to express himself and herself anew, uniquely.

My own learning and putting together of discoveries over the last ten years has been exciting. Some aspects have also been painful, difficult and slow to reveal themselves.

This third edition is written out of this background, and will inevitably be coloured by it. I can only hope that readers may take it as an encouragement to follow their own journey into helping and counselling.

I would particularly like to thank Sarah V. Smith, Senior Editor at Baillière Tindall, for her continued warm and enthusiastic support and challenge. My thanks also to Margaret Wellings for typing yet another manuscript. And a thank you to the countless people who, in courses and workshops, have sharpened my perceptions and unwittingly helped me understand something I was trying to teach. A thank you also to those who trusted themselves to my counselling efforts; that is where most of the real learning happens.

Verena Tschudin

1 'Charity begins at home'

The counsellor in you

'Know thyself' is one of the oldest dictums in history. But do you know yourself?

The more you are aware of yourself, the more you are aware of other people. Awareness of other people and their strengths and needs in turn helps you to be aware of these things within yourself. This is the basis of all helping, be this making a person comfortable in bed; to come to terms with illness or suffering; or to find ways of living more appropriately.

Counselling and helping is only possible from a basis of self-awareness and insight into how people live and work, think and feel. This is not just book-knowledge, but real, raw knowledge of who you are and what you are about.

Today, there are many ways of developing insight about oneself. From psychoanalysis, astrology, intelligence tests, psychometric tests, the Myers–Briggs Type Indicator and Chinese horoscopes, to quick self-assessments in magazines and books, there is a great wealth of information available on how to understand oneself better.

Any measurements which 'reveal' ourselves are only partial. They are never the truth, the whole truth and nothing but the truth. The greatness, and also the difficulty, of self-awareness is that there is always more to a person or a situation than can be known or predicted.

As we go through life we grow and develop, and new aspects constantly occur. Self-awareness is therefore a never-ending experience. To understand our basic temperament can indeed be very helpful and may remove much pain and guilt, and allow the development of a natural assertiveness. But beyond that, we are what we allow ourselves to be. In this way we discover not only ambiguities and discrepancies, but we also discover meaning and purpose.

As you allow yourself to sit and stare, and take time to be aware of yourself, you are laying the basis for being a counsellor. Counselling is not about giving the right answer, but it is about being with another person 'there where it hurts'. That means that you have a sense of that hurt because you have experienced something similar. It does not mean identifying with another, but going alongside.

Gilmore (1973) believes that a lack of self-understanding means that there are areas about ourselves that are unknown to us. What we don't know about ourselves we tend not to acknowledge in others, and thus we reduce our capacity for helping. When we increase our self-understanding, we increase our capacity to help.

Awareness is not something which we learn from books. Insights and flashes of inspiration may come from books, but having an awareness of oneself is a way of life. Marson (1979) says:

> To be aware of one's own deep feelings and to be able to understand and predict one's own emotional responses leads to greater self security.

Awareness of ourselves is strengthening, and gives us control and the freedom to be that which we really are.

A 'portrait of a helper'

The more we are ourselves, the more real we are as *people* generally, not only as helpers.

Egan (1982) describes some of the characteristics of people who are or want to be helpers. These are of course general traits, and every helper fits into such a 'portrait' uniquely. Helpers, he says, are:

> first of all committed to their own growth – physical, intellectual, social-emotional, spiritual – for they realize that helping often involves modelling the behavior they hope others will achieve. They know they can help only if, in the root sense of the word, they are 'potent' human beings – that is, people with both the resources and the will to act ... They have common sense and social intelligence ... They know that the fruit of listening lies in effective responding ... They will draw on all possible helping resources that will enable their clients to achieve their (the clients') goals ... They follow a comprehensive helping model, but they

are not rigid in its application. The model is not central; clients are. The model is an instrument of helping clients live more effectively ... Skilled helpers have their own human problems, but they do not retreat from them. They explore their own behaviour and know who they are.

You do not become a good helper only after you have acquired all the skills. You do not have to be perfect in theory before you can help anybody. You learn by doing, and doing teaches you.

What portrait do you have of yourself as a helper? What are your reasons for wanting to learn about counselling and helping skills? You have often helped people in this way; what did *you* get out of it?

When you realize that you want to use counselling, not because you are good at it but because through counselling some deep need within yourself is satisfied, then you are sincere and genuine, and that comes across to the person who is helped. This is not to say that you are an unfulfilled person, but that you have recognized and acknowledged your own needs and respond to them in the most adequate way for you yourself. When you know your true needs, and what makes you tick, then you are more free to listen to others. Or, as Rogers (1961) said:

One way of putting this ... is that if I can form a helping relationship to myself – if I can be sensitively aware of an acceptant toward my own feelings – then the likelihood is great that I can form a helping relationship toward another.

Self-awareness goes together with certain attributes which are essential to helping. In a sense you have to 'be' these things to yourself before you can be them to and with others.

Genuineness   Most writers and teachers about counselling and helping have written about three essential elements in that process: genuineness, warmth and empathy. The helper 'only' needs these three traits, or characteristics, and bingo!, helping takes place.

Helping *is* that simple. Genuine helping happens when these elements are there. But to *be* any of these things genuinely is not easy. Helping is not a set of skills, but a way of being, as Rogers (1980) repeatedly said.

Rogers also used the words 'congruence' and 'realness' for the same thing. It means a coming-together of experience and awareness and communication.

Experience drove home the fact that to act consistently acceptant, for example, if in fact I was feeling annoyed or skeptical or some other non-acceptant feeling, was certain in the long run to be perceived as inconsistent or untrustworthy. I have come to recognize that being trustworthy does not demand that I be rigidly consistent but that I be dependably real. The term 'congruent' is one I have used to describe the way I would like to be. By this I mean that whatever feeling or attitude I am experiencing would be matched by my awareness of that attitude. When this is true, then I am a unified or integrated person in that moment, and hence I can *be* whatever I deeply *am*. This is a reality which I find others experience as dependable. (Rogers, 1961)

To be consistent in a helping relationship demands many of the skills described later. It also asks of you as helper that you use all the communication skills at your disposal. But more than that, consistency of behaviour denotes a large measure of self-awareness. When you know yourself, then you are less likely to be put off, found out, or be dishonest with others. It demands awareness of yourself, but it also demands that you share that awareness in the relationship. Nurse (1980) puts this into context:

When we are at our place of work, occupying a particular position in a social structure, it is all too easy to take refuge in our professional role as tutor, midwife, nursing officer or whatever it may be, and to use that role as a means of protecting ourselves or as a substitute for effectiveness.

It is possible to take refuge in a perceived role: that of being kind, or caring or just. These may be acceptable ways of being, and they are very good ones, but only if they are 'real' to the person concerned. When you are able to identify the discrepancies in your life, particularly those which affect your abilities to help others, then you become a more genuine, more consistent person.

When I am 'in-place', there is a reasonable convergence between my professed values and how I actually live, between how I think and how I actually live, between how I see my behaviour from inside and how it looks to others from outside. My living testifies to what my values are. To the extent that there is significant division between inner and outer, I am not wholly in my actions; I am divided within myself, and in the end must be uncertain who I am and what I am about. (Mayeroff, 1972)

Only when you are not trying to be 'somebody' but are simply yourself can you be trustworthy, dependable and consistent, and only then will you be seen as such by the client.

Warmth

This character trait of helpers has also been described in many ways: 'non-possessive warmth' and 'unconditional positive regard' are perhaps the best known.

Rogers (1980) cites a study done with teachers and students where it was found that teachers who got the best out of their students had high levels of self-regard, disclosed themselves to the students, responded to their feelings and ideas, gave them praise, and 'lectured' less often.

The teachers had a high regard for themselves. They didn't show off, but somehow knew their place in the world and felt at home in it. Therefore they could share, listen, praise, and not feel threatened or throw their weight around. They worked hard and played hard. They came across as genuine people.

Being warm does not necessarily mean being effusive, particularly if this is not your style or normal way of behaving. It does mean respecting another person, and what that person is and stands for.

This warmth is described as non-possessive, or unconditional. This is not easy. We all have our own agendas and, particularly as nurses, we are used to giving advice and telling people what to do. This kind of warmth does not lecture, but gives of itself.

The next sections elaborate upon this characteristic.

Accepting

You can often hear phrases like 'I can accept him making unreasonable demands on me when he is tired, but I cannot accept that he smacks the children'.

One cannot accept someone piecemeal: 'This bit of you is OK but this bit is not'. We may not like what we encounter, but a person is all of a person, warts and all.

It is almost impossible to be totally acceptable; few people are that aware or that saintly. Accepting means, however, that we become ever more aware of ourselves in order to be more aware of others.

Accepting another person without judgement may occasionally seem incredible to a client. Someone who has lost self-esteem sees the world through the eyes of that loss. To have someone who is accepted unconditionally is so opposed to this image that it may seem incredible, even ridiculous. It is then that the genuineness of the helper's character comes through: as a constancy of behaviour. Eventually the client just has to believe it with the result that it may provide the basis for self-acceptance.

Respecting

To be respectful is one of the fundamental characteristics of helpers: Egan (1982) says further, in his portrait of a helper:

> They respect their clients and express this respect by being available to them, working with them, not judging them, trusting the constructive forces found in them, and ultimately placing the expectation on them that they do whatever is necessary to handle their problems in living more effectively.

Rogers (1967) says that

> the therapist communicates to his client a deep and genuine caring for him as a person with potentialities, a caring uncontaminated by evaluations of his thoughts, feelings, or behavior.

How do you respect yourself? If in a fit of either self-pity or exultation you eat a box of chocolates all at once, do you respect this act, or feel guilty about it? Respecting yourself has something to do with assertion; not standing on a soap-box, but knowing what is there, and not denying it.

Trusting

Trusting means having confidence or faith in someone or something. A boat-builder on a desert island would trust himself to escape unharmed once he had built a safe boat. Another person good at gardening or cooking might be more likely to survive on the island by being properly fed. These people would trust themselves and their abilities and skills even under difficult circumstances. What skills and abilities do you have in which you trust? Are there other areas in which you trust in yourself?

In a crisis, many (perhaps most) people lose a certain amount of their confidence in themselves. They then need to trust in someone else to help them through such a crisis. Thus patients trust a doctor to help them get better; they trust the nurse to deal competently with their infusions; they trust friends not to talk about their home situation in the pub; they trust helpers to make an effort to understand them.

As nurses we are often in a position to be trusted by our patients. This puts us in a privileged position. It means that we have the patient's confidence even before we do any work with him. In turn, we trust patients and their ability to cope. Our role as nurses is often one of coping, taking over, looking after the helpless, taking responsibility, and acting on behalf of patients (see p. 142) who are in need of our particular skills and on which their lives often depend. Yet even in illness and difficulty, patients, like children, are very robust. We need to trust that they not only can but will cope, whatever that entails. As a helper you should be sure that you are not

like the father who 'cares' too much and 'over-protects' his child and who 'does not trust' the child, and whatever he may think he is doing, he is responding more to his own needs than to the needs of the child to grow. (Mayeroff, 1972)

Trusting may mean actively giving patients permission to take responsibility for themselves as individuals, and then encouraging and reinforcing this again and again. It may also mean trusting patients' own judgement of themselves and their particular situation. For instance, at some point a patient may refuse to have any more treatment, in the knowledge that there are different ways of coping with disease which may differ from that of the doctor or nurse's expectations. This is not easy to accept as it implies a rejection of your skills and the care which you have given. At such a point you may have to ask, what is happening here? Is it a *rejection* of *your* skills and available know-how, or is it an *affirmation* of your client's own person? If it is the latter, then your skills have actually helped your client, but perhaps not in the way you had expected. Accepting a client's decision may indeed be the proof of effective helping.

Caring

> In the sense in which a man can ever be said to be at home in the world, he is at home not through dominating, or appreciating, but through caring and being cared for. Mayeroff (1972)

The *Oxford English Dictionary* defines 'to care' as meaning to 'feel concern or interest; feel regard, deference, affection'. It is certainly that, but it is also much more. Caring is 'the human mode of being' says Roach (1987); it is 'humankind at home, being real, being his or herself'.

Caring, like its grammatical root-word charity, begins at home. Caring is not a duty, nor a survival technique, nor even a skill. Caring is that which characterizes us as human beings.

Roach elaborates her statement by saying that caring is made up of five Cs: compassion, competence, confidence, conscience and commitment. Compassion is seen as an awareness of a person's relationship with all living creatures. Competence is the knowledge, skill, experience and energy a person brings to professional work with others. Confidence is, according to Roach, the quality which fosters trusting relationships. Conscience is a moral awareness – the compass which directs a person's behaviour (see p. 140) – born out of experience and tested in relationships. Commitment is a choice made out of an awareness of desires and obligations.

'We are by nature to be for others', says Roach (1985) elsewhere. When we care for others, then we are also cared for. Mayeroff (1972) goes on:

> In a meaningful friendship, caring is mutual, each cares for the other: caring becomes contagious. My caring for the other helps activate his caring for me; and similarly his caring for me helps activate my caring for him, it 'strengthens' me to care for him.

Or, as Speck (1978) describes it practically:

> A young patient, who had suffered with leukaemia for several years, was readmitted to hospital. The ward staff knew her and her family very well, and were therefore upset when she eventually died on the ward. On the day when the patient died, the nurse in charge was a person who had formed a strong attachment to

the patient and her husband since they were of a similar age group and had several interests in common. Immediately after the death, the nurse in charge attended to the patient and then went into the office, sat down, and wept. The patient's husband followed her into the office and said to her, 'You looked after her well and did all that could be done. Don't upset yourself so – I'll fetch you a cup of tea'.

Caring is mutual; it is reciprocal. When you give, you receive, somehow. But you don't give in order to get. That is the difference between helping – caring – and most other transactions. That is why helping and caring are so satisfying, and so elusive.

Feelings in the helper

The more you know yourself, the more intensely you feel and live, the more 'potent' you become. When you meet with someone in a helping relationship, not only do you feel for and with that other person, that person also arouses feelings in you. Some of these may be good, helpful feelings, and some may be difficult and not easy to deal with.

The following quotation was written about wars and revolutions. It can also apply to nursing.

Confrontation with human pain often creates anger instead of care, irritation instead of sympathy, and even fury instead of compassion. (Nouwen et al, 1982)

Strong emotions can be evoked in the face of someone else's suffering. When your emotions are roused in the face of suffering, you may not be able to help. You are too much aware of your own reactive suffering. To be truly human means at times to feel anger, irritation and fury in the face of suffering.

A client may arouse all kinds of feelings in you, from surprise to hope, from irritation to resentment. A rabbi wrote the following:

I learned that allowing yourself to be used and even misused on occasion is what living and eternal living is about. Everyone knows it who deals with such tricky creatures as human beings like us. (Blue, 1985)

You may also feel helpless and powerless with a patient. A conversation has started and you don't know how to continue it. You feel resentful at your own inability to cope.

You may be left with unfinished business in a helping relationship.

This patient, who was slowly dying, felt helpless in the face of his wife's handling of the domestic affairs and repeated often that he had to knock some sense into her. He is slipping away from me now, and I can't grasp him to knock sense into him. I can only feel the pain of never seeing the result of my help.

You may feel bewildered when a patient presents a problem which you may not understand, or which your moral, ethical or religious feelings question.

You may feel sexually aroused by and attracted to a patient. Or a patient may openly express sexual feelings towards you. This can cause indignation, guilt and annoyance on both sides.

Helping and counselling is based on *feelings*, and on the *person* who has feelings. You are helping that person within a relationship, therefore you are involved, and that means your feelings are important too. This goes right back to awareness, and to starting at home and first looking after yourself.

One of the caricatures of helping is the situation where a client says something like 'My whole world collapsed since I broke my arm', and the 'helper' replies, 'You should worry! When I broke my leg . . .'.

To help another person often means that you come across situations which ring bells for you, or touch a raw nerve in you. They put you in touch with a similar situation or feeling which you have never really 'worked through'. This is particularly common in situations of loss. Your patient only has to mention a parent's recent burial, and you are in touch with what happened to you when you lost one of your parents. There is nothing wrong with that; indeed if it didn't happen, it would be more alarming. What *is* difficult is if you are then so much 'into' your own feelings that you can't help, and your client becomes helper to you. And yet, helping *is* reciprocal. You are helped by your client. The crunch is *how* you are helped.

When you know yourself and your feelings, then you can use them to help yourself and others. When you don't know them, then you will be surprised when they pop up at the most unexpected moments, and then they tend to be out of hand and destructive. Take time to make friends with yourself and your feelings!

Beliefs and values

One of the 'five Cs' is conscience. Like feelings, conscience needs to be known and used in the right way. Like your feelings, your beliefs and values show themselves to others, even though you may not be aware of it.

Ethics is an area of life which is coming more and more into the public debate, and rightly so. You need to know where you stand, and from what basis you care and help. This is nowhere more topical than in the concept of primary nursing. You are a more autonomous nurse in this type of work than ever before.

Your beliefs and values will therefore colour your work and your relationships with patients, relatives and colleagues. Your attitude will quickly convey itself to all with whom you come in contact. Do you trust a patient, and on what grounds? Do you accept a patient, fleas and all? Do you respect your colleague, even though you consider her overweight, slovenly, or lazy? Do your prejudices colour your behaviour?

A patient may be talking with you about fears of dying, and the question of euthanasia comes up. You may have quite strong feelings about it. Do you feel that you have to be helpful, neutral, or influencing this person? How do you know that your views and beliefs are the right ones, or the better ones?

In helping and counselling there is a lot of listening to be done: to yourself and to your client. Sometimes you may not know what you believe; sometimes you may be very sure. Sometimes you may change completely in the course of a conversation. You may end up by being quite confused about your feelings and your conscience. This is uncomfortable, and quite common. A few lines ago I suggested that you make friends with your feelings; here I suggest that you make friends with your conscience. Helping is not giving the other person your point of view, but helping individuals to listen more carefully to their own being and to find the right answer there.

Any situation of change or learning begins with the now, the given. When it comes to self-knowledge, most of us know ourselves very little, perhaps out of fear, perhaps out of neglect.

Helping is not one-sided. It is involved, and involving. You can only help someone out of your own self, your own understanding and out of what you have got. It is therefore not only right, but also a duty, to know yourself, to start with yourself, to love yourself.

2 Support systems

Why support is needed

As charity begins at home, so does support. Before anyone can support another person, he or she needs to be supported.

Support is not something which is always readily available in nursing, although in recent years it has come to be more appreciated and increasingly available. The prevailing culture in nursing is still largely that nurses should not get 'involved' or 'emotional' about difficult situations (Moore, 1984), should be able to sort out their own feelings (Knight, 1979), or are strong anyway (otherwise they shouldn't be nurses) and have learnt early to cope with their own feelings (Raeburn, 1979).

It is significant that as long ago as 1972 the Committee on Nursing (Briggs Report) listed some of the topical reasons why nurses should have support:

The changing nature of medical care has added to the strain imposed on nursing and midwifery staff – anxiety about errors in medicine dosage, fears of machinery, the constant tension in intensive care units, the ethical problems of abortion, transplantation and resuscitation, uncertainty over rapid decisions to be made in times of crisis, the care of an increasing number of patients with mental disorders.

To this list, written almost 20 years ago, must now be added the constant reorganizations of work, increasing shortage of staff, increased requirements for documentation, uncertainty over grading and, with the introduction of Project 2000, completely new ways of working and learning.

The culture in which nurses work contributes greatly to some of the pressures they experience. The work done by Menzies and her subsequent report (1960) highlighted many of the destructive practices which existed in nursing at that time 'as a defence against anxiety'. Much has changed since then, and much has not. 'Defence' is still more often the working model than awareness, and 'attack' is more common than facing the problem.

Daily contact with patients and illness enables nurses to talk easily about issues which are taboo for most people: death, illness, facing diminishment and acquired immune deficiency syndrome (AIDS), to mention just a few. To go with a person into these realms is like constantly overstepping conventionally accepted boundaries; this cannot be done without cost.

The combination of emotional giving and management pressure is a potent force which may push nurses to the brink and cause them to 'burn out'.

On the whole, nurses are not particularly kind, generous and supportive of each other. It is astonishing how we can be regarded as 'angels' to patients but often just the opposite to colleagues. It is perhaps not surprising therefore that many ways of support are still theoretical rather than practical.

The support systems available

There are many possibilities of, and for, support. I will first outline five classical possibilities.

Counsellors

A counsellor for the staff, and for nurses in particular, can be the most valuable support. This is for three reasons: a counsellor can give clients the safety to explore their real feelings, and the permission to talk about the things which are of the utmost importance to them, particularly the knowledge that they have been heard (Crawley, 1983). So that there is indeed 'safety' for a client, a counsellor needs to be completely independent, i.e. not attached to a school or college of nursing, or to administration, either in salary or in the location of the office. Where these criteria apply, Jones (1978) suggests, from a survey of student nurses, that 98% would use the service.

Groups

The next important area of support is *groups*. Most people need to talk to other people in order to feel appreciated. Seeing that others have the same needs and problems is invaluable, and this cannot be learnt in isolation, hence the need for a group.

Such support groups for nurses can deal with issues related particularly to work, such as professional identity, techniques for stress management, methods of conflict management, how to increase staff members' sense of self-esteem and self-confidence, while at the same time increasing their knowledge of and skill in nurse–patient interactions (Scully, 1981).

To be effective, support for nurses needs to be continuous, and groups are the most perennial form of giving support; they are flexible in time, context, content and style. But support groups will only function well if they have an aim, if they are oriented towards action and towards a specific goal, although this may be a changeable goal. A group which meets solely for the sake of meeting may not be successful, unless that is its specific goal. Groups may be used for a limited period only, or may persist. The membership may change, but any changes should be discussed and implemented, not just allowed to happen, otherwise the group will disintegrate.

Occupational health departments (OHDs)

Seen as part of an overall supportive environment, staff in OHD 'can advise an employee on how to improve and maintain health, or prevent occurrence of ill-health or injury. Employees can also voluntarily seek advice about much broader problems connected with personal, social, work or economic factors' (Clark, 1978).

Many problems become large because there is no one available to listen. When the problem has been heard and shared, it is often halved in magnitude. OHDs are one possible setting for lending an ear.

Education

A strong area of support for nurses is *education*. Nurses need to be skilled not only in nursing activities, but also in human activities. Learning about counselling should not simply be a matter of buying a book; it should also include teaching in the health care environment.

Any nurse can stick a needle or an enema into anything human and, for that matter, into beings which are not human. But not all nurses can supply optimum care. (Jourard, 1971)

The education needs to be in the technique of giving optimum care. When nurses fail

to encourage patients to share their anxieties and to express their emotions ... it is seen that the nurses' motivation for withholding information is *not* that it is better for the patient, because he cannot cope with it; but that it is better for the nurse, because she does not know how to handle it. (Cox, 1979)

Systematic education should include such topics as stress and its management; personal and professional ethics, with particular reference to any speciality in which the nurses are working; supportive and interpersonal skills, such as helping and counselling; and leadership skills. When nurses are skilled in these areas, then they can give optimum care. When we do that, then

our practice (is) concerned with humans and is humanizing ... Titles bestowed on us by organizations do not give us the authority to be effective in practice. That authority comes only through sound knowledge. (Partridge, 1978)

Many of these aspects are part of the curriculum of Project 2000. Nurses not trained in that mode, and that is still the majority of nurses at present, need particular help and training.

Co-counselling
Co-counselling is a way in which nurses can support and help each other. It needs no external organization, money or resources. Co-counselling is a

reciprocal method of counselling whereby two people meet to take turns as client and counsellor, using specific skills known to both. (Bond, 1979)

Co-counselling looks specifically at the areas of hurts from the past or present life. It enables one to identify these areas, to own or disown areas of the personality, and to uncover areas which had either been repressed or allowed to lie dormant. In doing so it has enabled people who use it to increase their ability to relax, think more clearly, re-evaluate and re-structure beliefs which might now be seen to be outdated, change behaviour patterns, increase emotional warmth towards others, and control their own emotional outbursts.

The technique, as the word co-counselling suggests, is carried out in pairs. Each person should have the same or similar skills. It should be organized so that each person takes an equal amount of time to be client and helper. This may be half an hour each, or an hour each per week, alternating. How it is organized does not matter, as long as it is equal and one person is not always giving and the other always receiving the support.

The next important element is that each member of the pair chooses beforehand how much help is wanted from the helper. This may not be the same for each member of the pair at the same session. One person may want the helper mainly to listen, another may look for the use of a particular skill from the helper; yet another may want help with keeping to the process. No pair of co-counsellors will work in the same way or get the same results, but

sometimes skills buried for years or not known about at all, emerge and become available to the person. And, whatever else it may or may not do, co-counselling does train a person to be a careful and unique listener. (Townsend and Linsley, 1980)

Supervision

Supportive, competent supervision is essential if nurses are to give their best to the care of the ill, frail and vulnerable. (Ogier and Cameron-Buccheri, 1990)

Yet what supervision *is* is not very clear to most nurses. Some helping agencies have defined supervision as having three main functions:

1. A management function.
2. A support function.
3. A training and staff development function.

Supervision gives rights and responsibilities to both parties. The supervisor should ensure that the supervisee is aware of policies, has an adequate workload, has the tools available to carry out the work; that the work is fairly evaluated and this is communicated to the supervisee; and that the supervisee is supported, particularly during stressful times.

The supervisee on the other hand is accountable (see p. 144) to the supervisor for the work done and the way it is carried out.

Both parties are responsible for seeing that supervision takes place on a regular basis. Together they should determine the supervisee's developmental needs, and both should agree how these will be met.

Heywood Jones (1989) tells of a health visitor with considerable experience who also showed enthusiasm and innovative practice in a new post. Her difficulty was that she did not keep her secondary records up to date. She was aware of this and had asked for help by requesting her manager to ask for the records on a regular basis. This help was not forthcoming and the health visitor was finally brought before a professional conduct committee, accused of fifteen charges concerning documentation.

This incident illustrates several factors already alluded to:

a) The pressure of work.
b) The pressure of documentation.
c) The pressure to be innovative.
d) Lack of supervision.
e) Lack of personal support (she knew her weak spot but was not helped to change).
f) The inability to deal with the problem in a supportive way, using punishment instead.

On a practical level, Ogier and Cameron-Buccheri (1990) found that supervision was more satisfactory when it was supportive rather than controlling. This meant mainly asking open questions (see p. 80), rather than checking: 'Have you done ... ?'

Sometimes there is a need to talk to someone about a particular patient, but it is impossible to do so to a colleague or a senior member of the team because of issues of confidentiality. A supervisor is then not only the ideal but also the appropriate person. Jacobs (1982) suggests that

particular anxieties which many counsellors have are about handling feelings of love, aggression, sexuality and power. Training for (pastoral) counselling requires some mastery of the anxiety about such feelings, whether they are shown by clients, or are seen in different forms in counsellors themselves.

These are not issues which can be solved in a few minutes, and cannot be talked about to just anybody. Therefore supervision which is ongoing, supportive and challenging is essential.

Who should be a supervisor is an essential question. Ideally it should be a person of experience who has insight into the supervisee's work. This may be another nurse, but not one from the same unit or department as the supervisee.

Some supervision is possible in groups, either outside the working environment or in a support group. The support given by a whole team to a particular patient may be discussed, and different styles and approaches examined. The issue of confidentiality needs to be kept in mind and respected.

Groups can be very useful, and indeed powerful, sources of supervision. Forms of self-sharing by all the members of the group can lead them to see where the wider issues in dealings with clients might be improved.

Which support should you have?

Because of the various pressures under which nurses work, support is often a question of 'yet one more thing'. Or a manager says that you can have support, but only as one possibility from among others. The different areas outlined above do not in any way constitute all the possibilities. Nurses who have felt strongly enough that they need support have used all manner of ways to get it. They meet in the pub at lunchtime once a fortnight; they meet in each other's houses; they ask a social worker or chaplain to supervise a few of them in a group; they use friends as counsellors; they pass books and articles around on specific topics of mutual interest. Some area health authorities have funded innovative projects where counselling is available within a setting of advice and information. There are peripatetic counsellors. Others have set up help-lines for colleagues in similar work. There are numerous examples in industry of workers providing their own support if management were slow in producing proposals. There are equally numerous examples, documented in the nursing press (e.g. Hancock, 1983; Pembrey, 1987; Swaffield, 1988; Jesson and Wilmot, 1990), of the need for support and what some nurses have done about this need both individually and in groups.

That there is a need for support is not in dispute. The support you give to your patients does, however, reflect the support you get. All nurses strive to give their patients all the support necessary; it is ironic, therefore, that they should often have to fight so hard to get even the basic support for themselves. The more enlightened types of management have recognized that their staff work better if they are well cared for in their work. Supportive activities should be encouraged by every means possible. We do not need just a National Health Service; it should also be a healthy service.

Support in nursing is greatly lacking, but at the same time, more and more nurses are aware of their need for support, and look for it and create it among themselves. There are traditional and spontaneous forms of support; there are those which an institution should supply and those which an individual should go out and get. At any one time, one form may be more appropriate than another; it should not be a question of either/or, but of this *and* that. Only a supported nurse can give optimal care.

3 The context of counselling

Disease and illness

The counselling and helping done by nurses is unique in that it takes place within the context of physical illness and pain, but, as every nurse knows, this is only the shell or the obvious and practical side of helping. What cannot be so easily seen and touched is just as real: the suffering within the person who is ill. With more and more emphasis on holistic care and primary nursing, it is clear that both these aspects need to be taken into account. Salvage (1990) cites research which found that 'patients judged the quality of nursing by its emotional style', that is, by the nurses' awareness of patients' practical and *emotional* needs, and their response to both.

The patient may be very ill and unable to be either totally or partially self-caring, becoming a passive recipient of care without the ability to express any emotions, but still feeling more than just a body to be cared for.

Other patients may simply have to be 'serviced': a quick operation and some stitches to be removed; or a delivery without any complications.

For most patients though, illness and disease is 'a moment of truth'. Even an appendicectomy can bring into focus some aspect of that person's life which he had never thought about. Most illness brings with it a kind of loss: a loss of health, of an organ, of time, of relationships, of mobility or life-style. This generally concerns not only the patient or client, but the family, friends and many others who are significant in that person's life. Most of us go through life with an attitude of 'It won't happen to me' and, when it does happen, the moment of truth can be quite shattering. It needn't be a big blow, like an accident or cancer. Having your bunions done is just as often a trigger for facing that 'It *has* happened to me'. An external event is the vehicle for internal searching and adjustment. When, as a nurse, you show to a patient that you are aware of these possibilities and take them into account whilst discussing them, your style becomes 'emotional' and the patient responds favourably.

Some of the aspects of this emotional care are discussed in this chapter. But these are merely the obvious points against a backcloth of all human life which is exposed in hospitals and sickrooms. Not only are people different, but cultures are different; beliefs, backgrounds and experiences are different; and they all greatly influence how a patient will act and react to any given situation. Perhaps the main thing that can be said is that, with respect for the individual, real help is possible.

The relationship between nurses and patients

All helping and counselling is done within a relationship. In nursing, that relationship already exists, in that every patient is looked after by at least one if not more nurses. The way you use that relationship is therefore of paramount importance.

Be aware for a moment how your contact with a patient starts:

1. The patient is sick; the nurse is healthy.
2. The patient is needy; the nurse can fulfil the need.
3. The patient has only the nurse to relate to; the nurse has other patients and colleagues if she needs a break.
4. The patient is dependent, the nurse has power.
5. The patient is lying down, the nurse is standing over him or her.
6. The patient may have needs of intimate bodily care, and the nurse, a stranger, gives it without question.

This list makes it quite clear that the relationship which a nurse and patient have is basically a very unequal one: one has, the other has not. This is true of many other situations but the inequality is often reduced, in that the one who needs a service pays for it. The two partners thus become more equal. In nursing, this is impossible.

The relationship based on power and authority (the 'doctor [nurse] knows best' attitude, with an active nurse and passive patient) has all but disappeared. However, remnants still exist; perhaps the closest to that model is the care given in emergencies and in intensive therapy units.

Salvage (1990) has pointed out that the 'new nursing' is based on a different kind of relationship between nurses and patients: that of partnership. This is a more creative relationship for both parties. It is one which also challenges. Given the unequal starting point of a nurse–patient relationship, partnership has to be worked on and established by negotiation.

In this kind of helping relationship there is no clear distinction between physical care and psychological care. One generally leads to the other, and they overlap and interact. A diabetic patient on a special diet needs advice about it; but she may also need to discuss fears about her future, her children's future, what this disease means to her, or any other aspect of life which is important to her. The challenge to the nurse is to deal with the *person*, not just her problems.

Regression

Attitudes towards illness and people who can help one to get better are learnt in childhood. When a person becomes seriously ill, this attitude is triggered into action and a grown person can behave like a child. Some children seek attention by 'being good' and submissive; others gain what they need by crying, moaning or complaining (Altschul and Sinclair, 1981) (see p. 108).

Mathews (1962) notes that

adult hospital patients, because of their fright and insecurity in the situation, regress to a child-like dependency and continuously seek reassurance. At the same time, however, this dependent status sets up a deep conflict within patients in their attempts to maintain the self-image as an adult. Patients react strongly against threats to their individuality, maturity and adulthood.

Nurses who are aware of such behaviour are more likely to deal sympathetically with patients, rather than dismissing it or playing the game with them. The notion of a partnership addresses the adult behaviour in patients, and this can in itself be therapeutic because it allows them to be, and be seen as, responsible.

Fear

A person's reactions to most situations of threat to individuality, maturity or survival is either fear or anger.

If we were to set down in order of importance the diverse feelings of our patients, fear would lead them all. Fear, perhaps the most powerful of all emotions, can give rise to behaviour over which patients have little or no control. (Burton, 1979)

Fear is a remarkably strong influence in everyone's life. Faced with anything unusual, we are afraid, and not just a little. When we are afraid, we generally fear 'the worst'. The woman who has discovered a lump in her breast fears 'the worst', that it is cancer, and her mind leaps to the thought 'death'. The person in an accident who has badly broken a leg fears 'the worst', that the leg might have to be amputated, and the mind leaps to 'my life ruined'.

Once the identity is threatened, we can become quite unable to handle simple, otherwise ordinary situations. We believe that everything is working against us. Fear creates fear, and a spiral of fear leads us to irrational behaviour. 'The only thing we have to fear is fear itself', said President Roosevelt, and not unjustly.

Fear tends to be a threat of danger to survival:

I won't make it.

This is a fear of physical survival, but it is also a fear of emotional survival.

I won't come through this operation.
I am no good as a woman any more.
I fear pain, therefore I won't have this test.
I feel I can't cope; don't ask me to help.
I don't trust myself; I always make a fool of myself.

Gilbert (1989) has described the basic mechanisms of defence as a 'go–stop process'. Fear leads more often to 'stop', and anger to 'go'. The behaviours and reactions arising out of fear are the helplessness and hopelessness so often seen in patients, and the paralysing inability to take any rational decision.

Anger and hostility

Anger is a common reaction to attack, be this attack by another person or an illness. What cannot be handled calmly and assertively gets the angry treatment.

Egan (1977) says that 'often the best defense is a good offense, and so people lash out before they can be attacked themselves'. Burton (1979) makes much the same point by saying that a fight reaction may be exactly what the words imply: hostile, resentful, belligerent ways which may or may not involve physical activity. Gilbert (1989) calls this the 'go' part of the process of defence, and in nursing it is known as 'fight': the time when the adrenalin rises.

Physical aggression may lead to injury, as it is meant to 'kill' the threat. 'Hostility includes the raging violence which results in cruelty and destruction' (Burton, 1979). She believes that few people recognize how hostile they can in fact be. Nurses are often the first in line of an attack by a patient, but doctors, radiographers, porters and ambulance crews may also be attacked. Such behaviour is normal when it is seen as part of a pattern of adjustment. When the anger has blown over, such a person will often recognize where it came from, and will realize that the extent of personal involvement is not only the 'other's' fault.

Nurses need to recognize that their professional standards may not be the same as other people's standards, and what they regard as a small matter and part of their work may spark off quite unexpected, hostile reactions in others.

Nurses who are on the receiving end of verbal or physical attack may take it personally and see it as a slight on their care-giving. This is not so. It is the client's problem: it is his fear, his uncertainty, his anger, his inability to cope. Physical attacks should never be condoned, but helping a person through anger is a challenge to anyone.

Shock

I collapsed at work on the Monday morning. I drove to work, walked across the car park and my left leg buckled underneath me; I couldn't stand. They took me to hospital and they did lots and lots of tests. They got Dr N to see me, and he said, 'Oh yes!', all bright and cheerful, 'you've got a tumour on the brain'. Well, that was a terrible shock. (Tschudin, 1981)

This patient had difficulty in believing that her left leg indicated that she had a tumour in her head. It would have been easier to believe that there was something wrong with her legs.

A Canadian patient in a taped interview told of her feelings after she heard she had cancer of the breast.

It did come as a tremendous shock to me, and to be quite honest, I didn't know whether to drive into an apartment or take a dip over Niagara Falls. My mind was in a terrible turmoil. (Walker, 1976)

Another patient told

how after some weeks of feeling unwell she woke up one morning realizing that her left side was paralyzed. She simply closed her eyes again and went to sleep for a few more hours.

The instinctive reaction to any bad news is 'oh no!'. The characteristic of shock is denial of what has happened: it can't be true.

The way in which this shock is expressed varies greatly. The patient who simply went to sleep again said that normally she never slept in. It may be a state of complete disorientation, or it may be the opposite: carrying on as if nothing had happened. Some cultures deal with shock by wailing and pulling out the hair. In shock, 'an abnormal reaction to an abnormal situation is normal' (Frankl, 1962).

Like physical shock, emotional shock will change and wear off. And, as with physical shock, a person who is emotionally shocked needs gentle handling. A shocked person will probably not hear anything spoken but what is 'heard' is the sensation of touch. Because such people are 'frozen', the warmth of close contact can be the most appropriate way to help them to come to the reality of the present. The 'unfreezing' happens when the person begins to talk. And then, like melting ice, the talking may be fast and abundant.

My husband had been in hospital after a heart attack – that was some years ago now, when they kept them in longer. He was getting on well and had phoned me to say he was feeling well. The next morning the nurse rang to say he had had a very bad night. I got to him an hour before he died. I stayed a bit but then went home and phoned the family, and A. who had been to see him last night. She was round like a shot. We sat on the sofa for a long time, not saying anything really but she was holding me like a child. Then I said something about it hurting. She put her arms around me more tightly and just said, 'it hurts, just there in the pit of the stomach, doesn't it'. I had never felt so completely understood as at that moment. I looked at her and as our eyes met I knew that everything would be alright.

Shock is a way of handling bad news of any kind. 'Tea and sympathy' has long been considered a standard remedy for this type of situation. While it has its limitations, this dictum has some validity.

Disbelief

In the process of adjustment to anything unexpected, such as illness, accidents, bereavement or loss of any kind, there is always a time of denial. The person who had a leg amputated still feels it clearly; the bereaved person still feels the missing partner in bed; when you have had something stolen you can still touch it. This is a normal phenomenon and a way in which the psyche or mind comes to terms with what happened. To cut oneself off all at once from something which had been essential to life seems impossible, therefore a time of disbelief is like a process of gradually letting go of what is now no longer there.

A mentally healthy person will be able to see this as a stage and work through it, going from an instinctive disbelief to an accepting and believing that it *did* happen, or *is* happening.

When disbelief turns into a more permanent mechanism of defence it becomes a denial of the past and the present. The patient is denying having cancer and tells her relatives and friends that the surgeon just took the breast off as a precaution. To counter such a statement with 'But you do have cancer' is not helpful because in that person's make-believe world there is no such thing as cancer. To see it as a coping or defence mechanism (see p. 110) would be more realistic, and could form the basis for giving help.

Misunder-standing

A very common defence mechanism of patients is that of not hearing what has been said, or hearing only what they want to hear or can cope with.

The doctor that I'm under, he's told me that he can cure me. At the start when I came down to London, they found that I had a small pancreas in the back of my head, and the fluid couldn't drain out at the other side and had stopped working. So they fitted a small pump and a tube that goes to a bag at the side of my bladder, that pumps it through so that the bladder is not overloaded. They also found this tumour which they said they can't get out by a normal operation, as under the knife. It could cause me to be paralysed, or could cause blindness, or something like that. But the doctor I am under now, he said they can cure it. They are treating my spine as well now so that the tumour separates the cells going down to my nervous system which could make me paralysed. So they can cure it now. (Tschudin, 1981)

This tale, from a taped interview, shows that the patient heard only what he could grasp. Some knowledge, some apprehension, an old wives' tale or two picked up somewhere, new and unusual surroundings, and the recipe for misunderstanding is complete.

Anyone who has ever asked for street directions will appreciate the problem. You may correctly hear the first direction or two, but then you get lost in right and left turns. You cannot cope with too much information when you are under stress, even the relatively minor stress of being lost in the street.

A patient may be nervous about seeing a doctor in the first place. He may have some questions to ask, but the doctor talks first. The doctor will probably use some medical terms of which the patient is unsure, but the patient is unwilling to appear ignorant. The apprehensive patient may have forgotten to switch his hearing aid on. Later, the doctor may say the same to his wife but when the patient and his wife get together, they have different stories.

It may only be a question of clarifying a word or technical term, or explaining a test or operation more fully. But, like denial, misunderstanding may have become a way of life and a permanent mechanism. The skill of helping is to see the difference and deal with it empathically.

Guilt

While anger blames the 'other', whatever or whoever it may be, guilt blames the self. A rule has been violated, and someone is responsible (Moorey and Greer, 1989). The 'rule' is often very deep rooted, and often also irrational. In order to make sense of a situation, most of us search for a reason and a meaning, and the conclusion may be so 'bad' that guilt is the only possibility.

Guilt feelings are always followed by a need for punishment. Being punished provides absolution, carrying with it the assurance that, although rejected for the 'bad' act which brought the guilt feelings, one may be restored to favour by paying for the act. There may be many ways in which adults 'ask for' punishment. If they are not punished by the environment in some way, by circumstances, or by other people, they will punish themselves. (Burton, 1979)

A reinforcing of guilt can happen when a patient believes he is infectious or 'dirty'. This is often a deep-seated feeling. Such patients may reject help of any kind, as they believe or imagine themselves to be outcast and beyond the reach of help.

Burton believes that it may not only be illness and accidents which lead to guilt, but that guilt feelings themselves can in fact cause illnesses and accidents.

Feelings of guilt and self-blame are very common in patients with cancers, or in their partners (King, 1984). It seems then that what matters is not so much whether this is a right or wrong interpretation by the patient, but rather whether it is helpful or harmful to the patient's recovery.

Shame

Shame is a kind of uncovering, appearing naked. According to Erickson (1964), shame can begin to appear in a child as early as the second year of life. During that year, a child becomes capable of independent action. If he fails at such actions, shame and doubt develop.

Shame is first of all an uncovering of ourselves to ourselves. 'A shame experience might be defined as an acute emotional awareness of a failure *to be* in some way' (Egan, 1986). The inadequacy is there, but unrecognized, until, because of some remark, happening or association, the inadequacy – the shame – is consciously recognized.

The area most often associated with shame is sexuality. We have learnt early to keep that subject under the duvet. Many people connect illness, particularly of the sexual organs, with wrongdoing in the past, with punishment, and with sin and guilt. They are ashamed of themselves for having such a disease. They imagine that the world around them will now find out or know about their wrongdoing. They feel that they should not or could not talk about their illness.

Such people suffer guilt in silence, giving thoughts, feelings and a negative imagination a stranglehold over them. It is all too easy to brush feelings of shame aside. 'Self-blame typically occurs in the absence of any other known or acceptable explanation' (King, 1984). Sometimes a simple explanation of anatomy can help a patient to see some illness or disease in perspective, where before he couldn't make a meaningful connection.

Feelings of shame can and need to be recognized and acknowledged. When they can be recognized, they can become valuable tools for growth and development.

The context in which counselling can and does happen is one of illness and disease. It is also one of much emotional searching and adjusting. Hospitals and sick-rooms are disturbing places. The symbol of an operation, of cutting and hurting in order to heal, is very powerful at all levels of care. It need not only be a 'real' operation which calls for counselling help; sometimes the more silent diseases of fear and guilt also need 'the sharp compassion of the healer's art' (Eliot, 1944).

4 The content of counselling

What is counselling?

What is counselling? This question must have been asked by everyone who has tried to help another person and each will probably have given a different answer.

In the last twenty years or so, the theory and practice of counselling have changed, and are still changing. It is useful to look at some definitions.

Any dictionary will probably define counselling as giving counsel or advice, or making recommendations. This is considered by those who counsel as being an inadequate definition, and even contrary to their practice.

Nurse (1978) cites some early definitions, among them one by J.H. Wallis: counselling is 'a dialogue in which one person helps another who has some difficulty that is important to him'.

The notes accompanying a BBC Radio 4 series on 'Principles of Counselling' give the following definition:

Counselling is . . . a way of relating and responding to another person, so that that person is helped to explore his thoughts, feelings and behaviour; to reach clearer self-understanding; and then is helped to find and use his strengths so that he copes more effectively with his life by making appropriate decisions, or by taking relevant action. Essentially then, counselling is a purposeful relationship in which one person helps another to help himself. (Inskipp and Johns, 1984)

The British Association for Counselling (BAC) has frequently rewritten its definition. The working definition adopted in 1989 may be rather lengthy, but it is also very comprehensive.

Counselling is the skilled and principled use of relationship to facilitate self-knowledge, emotional acceptance and growth, and the optimal development of personal resources. The overall aim is to provide an opportunity to work towards living more satisfyingly and resourcefully. Counselling relationships will vary according to need but may be concerned with developmental issues, addressing and resolving specific problems, making decisions, coping with crisis, developing personal insights and knowledge, working through feelings of inner conflict or improving relationships with others.

The counsellor's role is to facilitate the client's work in ways that respect the client's values, personal resources and capacity for self determination.

In BAC's *Code of Ethics* a shorter form is used:

The task of counselling is to give the 'client' an opportunity to explore, discover, and clarify ways of living more satisfyingly and resourcefully.

These varying definitions point to the fact that counselling is a complex task, involving 'exploring attitudes, values and beliefs about human nature, examining intentions and motivations, and exploring and learning ways of responding' (Inskipp, 1985).

The *task* of counselling is made up of various elements. Some of these are discussed below.

The relationship

Counselling needs two (or more) people: the client, and the helper. What is most important is the relationship they establish.

The goal of any helping profession is to provide growth, facilitating support and assistance (LaMonica and Karshmer, 1978). The three elements (the patient or client, the helper, and the relationship between them) have to be studied, understood, supported, and constantly evaluated. Counselling is not a one-way process, nor even a two-way process. It is a dynamic, circular or spiral process in which one element influences the other two, and they may never have quite the same influence twice.

In nursing we pay much attention to the patient or client, and rightly so. We pay much less attention to the helpers and their needs, and until recently we have almost neglected the relationship. By learning interpersonal skills, assertiveness and relaxation techniques, nurses are taking themselves as people and as professionals more seriously. However, so far it has rarely been accepted that patients really get better more quickly and more completely when they are cared for by a nurse with whom they get on.

When 'care' is translated into 'counselling', then the following quotation will sound very appropriate:

> If I can create a relationship characterized on my part
>   by a genuineness and transparency, in which I am
>   my real feelings
>   by a warm acceptance of and prizing of the other
>   person as a separate individual
>   by a sensitive ability to see his world and himself as
>   he sees them
> Then the other individual in the relationship
>   will experience and understand aspects of himself
>   which previously he has repressed
>   will find himself becoming better integrated, more
>   able to function effectively
>   will become more similar to the person he would
>   like to be
>   will be more self-directing and self-confident
>   will become more of a person, more unique and
>   more self-expressive
>   will be more understanding, more acceptant of others
>   will be able to cope with the problems of life more
>   adequately and more comfortably.
>
> (Rogers, 1961)

What Rogers is saying, and what the various definitions point to, is that the skills used in counselling are almost incidental. What matters is how the two people relate to each other. The skills of counselling *are* important, but that 'something other', those indefinable 'vibes', are just as important.

Skills

Counsellors could not call themselves 'experts' if there were not something in their repertoires which is extra to that which other people have. The skills *are* important (and half of this book is devoted to them), but they are there only for a wider, and further, purpose.

The process

Counselling exists so that the helped person can live more resourcefully and satisfyingly. For this to happen, three steps are necessary:

1. Defining the starting point; clarifying the problem.
2. Discovering a goal; getting to a 'better place'.
3. Exploring the ways and means of getting there.

Thus it is clear that counselling is goal oriented. It is not an analysis. But is is not *problem* oriented either. It is *person* oriented, intending to help the person with the problem. This means a flow, or movement forward, from one point to another; from dissatisfaction to satisfaction.

Self-help
Counselling is not 'doing for' the other. It does not prescribe. Counselling enables the client not only to solve a problem, but to be a more effective person, and that means knowing how to be effective. Self-help, or empowerment, are the outcomes of helping and counselling. This presupposes that 'when we treat people with the expectation that they will conduct themselves as healthy, attentive individuals, they generally do so' (Goldman and Morrison, 1984).

What counselling is not

It is easier to say what counselling is *not* than to say what it is. Giving advice, giving information, coaching, disciplinary interviews, guidance, recommending, per- suading, instructing and analysing are *not* counselling. Any of these activities may, however, lead to counselling.

The word counselling has crept into situations which are far from what the word means to a professional counsellor. This is true particularly, although not only, in nursing. 'I had to counsel her' is an oft-heard remark which reveals more about a manager's assumptions, and probable difficulty with interpersonal skills, than about the client's implied misdemeanour.

Nurses often have to give information, advice and guidance. They often have to instruct patients and colleagues in the use of equipment or techniques. They also often have to be counsellors. One of the skills of all 'helping' is to clarify issues, situations and relationships which are, or present, problems. By also being clear about what the method of helping is, the whole thing becomes easier. There is a sense in which 'calling a spade a spade' is truly helpful; both parties know where they stand with each other.

Giving advice, information or coaching is no less important, but by calling them 'counselling' they are not made more important. Each in its place could not be replaced by the other.

Counselling or helping? The unique function of the nurse, according to Henderson (1966) 'is to assist the individual, sick or well, in the performance of those activities contributing to health or its recovery (or to peaceful death) that he would perform unaided if he had the necessary strength, will or knowledge'.

These functions of a nurse surely include counselling. It is often claimed by professional counsellors that the counselling done by the 'helping professions' is simply part of their work and not *specifically* counselling. In particular, the aspects of contract (see p. 117) and payment are either absent or not so clear.

According to Nurse (1978), the helping which nurses do to fulfil their unique function falls into four parts:

1. Giving direct physical care.
2. Guide or advising.
3. Teaching.
4. Providing an environment which promotes the development of the individual in order to meet present or future needs.

A nurse cannot say that today only direct care will be given, or only provide the right environment. Without the one, the other is not possible; but it is only in the fourth of these activities that counselling, as such, can be seen to be possible. In the others, the nurse is helping, or caring.

Bowlby (1986) pictures a person in authority as 'someone walking more or less in the middle of a large band of people who are on the march . . . His caring task is to stay in touch with those in front and those behind, as well as those around him and to the sides, and to do all he can to prevent the whole band breaking into separate bits, or coming to a standstill and sitting down'.

Against this, Bowlby sees counselling as 'a one-to-one relationship which involves a mutuality of esteem . . . and the possibility of regular and sustained attention'.

I would argue that nurses have to be able to give care, help and counselling. They are expected to be experts in care. They are not expected to be experts in counselling, unless they are specifically employed as nurse counsellors. If you want to know when you care and when you counsel, you have to have a clear concept of yourself, your patient or client, and your relationship with that patient. It is often difficult to say when caring stops and counselling starts. Your awareness and skills are therefore of paramount importance. Both are necessary. I shall therefore continue to mention caring and counselling, and helping and counselling, together and interchangeably.

When is counselling suitable?

The counselling done by most nurses, except in mental illness, tends to be 'on the hoof'. This type of work is crisis oriented; it is short term and usually relates to a single issue. Out of this can, and sometimes do, come more contacts and more exploration. It is often the case that when one aspect of a person is examined and better understood, then other issues present themselves, also begging to be understood.

Quilliam and Grove-Stephenson (1990) give a list of statements which show the areas where counselling is most helpful.

I just want to be allowed to cry (get angry, feel afraid).
I need someone to listen to me.
I want to feel I'm OK.
I need someone to help me through.

This type of statement shows that the person needs *supportive* counselling.

I want to understand . . . .
I need to explore . . ..
I want to feel differently about . . . .
I want to clear up the confusion about . . ..

This type of remark shows that the patient or client is looking for some *insight* into his situation.

I want to act differently when . . ..
I'm not doing as well as I want to in . . . .
I need to change . . ..

These phrases show that the person is looking for *change* in his or her life.

In nursing, such statements are often not so neatly expressed. Statements like the following are more usual:

I don't know what's going on but I don't feel right.
I just can't make up my mind.
I want to help her, but I don't seem to get it right.

Helping someone by counselling means picking up

such opening remarks and following them through. Anyone who is in a situation, physically, mentally and spiritually, where he would rather not be, needs help. Very often it is difficult to know what the situation or problem actually is. It may be a practical problem, but if individuals are unable to solve a practical problem then they experience difficulties with the feelings involved, the mind-tracks or personal abilities and inabilities encountered. This is when another person helps by being alongside with counselling. Counselling, then, is either supportive of the person, helping an individual to gain insight, or to change an attitude.

The times and situations when counselling is unsuitable are probably few. People with a mental handicap are possibly not helped by counselling as such, although they need a great deal of care and attention. On the other hand, people with mental illness need a great deal of counselling. The type of help given here is more specific to the person's illness, and may also be given with clear guidelines and often on a one-to-one basis and in groups.

It may be that in your work you are asked to help a person by counselling, and that it fails. There may be many reasons for this, but undiagnosed mental illness may be one reason. When a patient's symptoms worsen or existing symptoms develop (Clarke, 1986), it is very likely that counselling has reached its limits and some more therapeutic help is needed.

Counselling may also be an inappropriate form of help for some people whose culture or religion deals with personal problems in an unfamiliar way.

For whom is counselling suitable?

In addition to those with a recognized psychiatric illness or mental handicap, most people can at times benefit from counselling. The psychologist Sigmund Freud believed that people near or above the age of 50 are not educable and that psychotherapy is not possible with them (Scrutton, 1989). This has been recognized as ageism, and Scrutton and others have done much to explode this myth.

That children need counselling just as much as adults is also being increasingly acknowledged. Reports of many forms of child abuse are increasingly heard and taken seriously. Counselling in this field is necessarily specialized and adapted to the world and understanding of children, although the basic concepts and theories still apply.

In your work as a nurse you will find many opportunities for caring and counselling. It is often in unexpected situations that help is most needed and most welcome: the patient who seems to cope well, but might just drop a hint that he has 'a little difficulty at home'; the person who had a colostomy and, on asking about his sex life, is told by the surgeon that there should be no problem, and who subsequently reveals to the nurse that he is homosexual (Wells, 1988); or the mother of a young baby who tells the health visitor that she thinks that her teenage step-daughter is taking drugs. These are unexpected situations, and perhaps one of the qualities nurses have to develop is a certain unshockability. More frequently, perhaps, the patient's problems are less unusual; or the nurse sees by the patient's behaviour or body language that there is something amiss.

Most counselling done by nurses is crisis oriented. Ideally, such work extends into developmental counselling. Once the immediate need for help is over, the person can begin to change. This is where more long-term help comes into its own. This may be difficult to achieve in the nursing setting, when patients are seldom cared for on a long-term basis. The ideal setting may be in the community, in rehabilitation areas, or in any situation of long-term care where patients must often make considerable adaptations in their attitudes to health and illness.

What counselling is can really only be experienced. As a nurse you may hesitate to call yourself a counsellor, but when you respond to a situation, then you are there as a person first and as a professional second, and the help you give may or may not be counselling. Whatever help you give, if it benefits the other person, it will have been appropriate.

5   *Theories of counselling*

Why have theories of helping?

It has often been said that all you need to do to help another person is listen. That is correct up to a point. If you know how to listen and what to listen for, you listen better.

Imagine that your client is in a place, emotionally and physically, where he or she would rather not be, although somewhere preferable may not be clear either. Your help clarifies this. It is then your responsibility as a helper or counsellor to enable your client to get from the present, uncomfortable position to the future, comfortable position. Helping is therefore something active. It is a process, a journey. Any journey is easier when you know how to do it. Many people have set out various theories and models for counselling, but they are eventually only different means of helping a person to change what needs to be changed.

Carl Rogers (1942) was the first to write about counselling. He talked about 'client-centred therapy'. In 1961, he wrote that 'jumbled sensings' had been the beginning. Rogers never produced a 'working model', remaining essentially a philosopher. Those who followed in his steps have put together different models and theories. These are generally problem management approaches.

When there is a framework, and when both helper and client know that framework, then the work done will be more focused, more satisfying, and possibly done more quickly. A framework is also useful for people who have little or no in-depth training, to help them to keep to the task. It is also useful for training people, particularly when 'stuck' or 'lost', to get back to a model and perhaps find a fresh perspective.

Table 5.1
Different
models for
helping

Egan	Carkhuff	Nelson-Jones
	Attending	
Problem definition		D Describe and identify the problem(s)
	Responding to clients	
		O Operationalize the problem(s)
	Personalizing the experience	
Goal development		S Set goals
	Initiating action	
Action		I Intervene
		E Exit and consolidate self-help skills

A model has to be simple to understand and simple to use. Nelson-Jones (1988) found that his trainees could not easily remember his model, but when he produced the acronym DOSIE (Table 5.1) they could remember the stages.

Just as each patient and client is different, so each helper is different. Which theory or model you use is eventually less important than that you use it confidently, and the client is helped effectively by it.

Different models

Table 5.1 shows three different approaches to helping. They are laid out in such a way that the reader can easily see where they coincide. It may also be helpful to compare these with the nursing process:

1. Assessment
2. Planning
3. Implementation
4. Evaluation.

Egan's model
Gerard Egan's model of helping (1986) has evolved and changed; he calls it 'a problem management approach to

helping'. He sees his three-stage model graphically as a circle, within which is another circle (evaluation) (Figure 5.1).

Stage 1: Problem definition. 'The client's problem situations and/or opportunities are explored and clarified.' This is the *present scenario*.
Stage 2: Goal development. 'Goals based on an action-oriented understanding of the problem situations are set.' This is the *preferred* or *future scenario*.
Stage 3: Action. 'Ways of accomplishing goals are devised and implemented.' *Getting the new scenario on line.*

Each of these three stages is further divided into substages, which also take the form of present scenario, future scenario, and getting the new scenario on line.

Although it is a non-directive approach, the helper is seen as someone who 'manages'. But the client 'manages' too. The helper can also be seen as a 'consultant', an expert, who negotiates with the client how to approach change, and to what end.

Egan sees counselling also as a 'social influence process': helping someone is always indirectly influencing his world. Counselling is therefore not just harmless talking, but powerfully responding to one's own environment and that of others. In this sense helpers, and eventually clients, need to possess the three elements of all skills: 'awareness, know-how, and assertiveness' (see p. 112).

Figure 5.1
Different models for helping

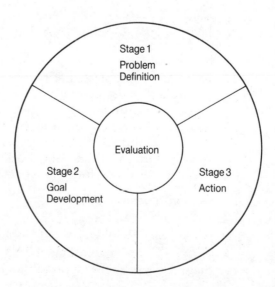

Carkhuff's model

Robert Carkhuff calls his theoretical approach a 'developmental model for helping' (1987). His basic premise is that 'to live is to grow'. Depending upon what we can do for ourselves, what others do for us, or what we do for others at crisis points in life is 'for better or for worse'. How we help at such crisis points is therefore crucial if it is to be for the better, i.e. for growing.

The three goals of helping, according to Carkhuff, are exploration, understanding and action. These combine in a process which recycles itself. Through action comes feedback, which leads to further exploration, and that in turn sets the stage for more accurate self-understanding. Into this setting come his four stages of helping: attending, responding, personalizing the experience and initiating action.

Attending is being with individual clients both physically and psychologically. We are with them verbally and non-verbally. The key ingredient of attending is listening.

Responding means hearing the client's words, but also being aware of behaviours and feelings. As these come to the fore, the helper responds, i.e. points them out, feeds them back to the client, makes them obvious and gives the client the possibility to see, hear and feel his or her ways of being.

Personalizing the experience is making the step from 'it happened because of . . .' to 'it happened because I . . .'. When the client is able to take responsibility for actions and feelings, then she will be more able to change because arbitrary forces are no longer working upon her, but she herself will make things happen. This can only be understood clearly when the client has seen the meaning and sense in these forces, and understands them in terms of herself or himself, i.e. personally.

Initiating action is the goal and also the first step along a new and different way of being. Carkhuff said that the goal is like the 'flip' side of the problem: when the problem is turned over, the goal is there! This is essentially what helping is about, and Carkhuff's model aims to do this by the above four steps.

Nelson-Jones' model

Richard Nelson-Jones (1988) intends that helper and client should collaborate to attain the goals at each stage of his 'model for managing problems'.

Stage 1: Describe. The task is to 'build a working alliance and help clients to reveal, identify and describe their problem(s)'.

Stage 2: Operationalize the problem(s). In this stage 'relevant information (for) defining and stating (the) problem(s) operationally' is gathered.

Stage 3: Set goals. Working goals should now be set and interventions negotiated to attain them.

Stage 4: Intervene. The task is now 'to lessen skills deficits and to build skills resources in problem area(s)'.

Stage 5: Exit. The process is reviewed and the helping relationship terminated only after the client has sufficient self-help skills in daily living.

Nelson-Jones bases his model on the premise that client self-responsibility is often a problem. Clients first of all need to be helped to own their problems, and then to acknowledge that they are responsible for what they do or fail to do to perpetuate their problems. It is his assumption therefore that clients need to develop the skills for coping with their problems. In that the helper adopts a problem management orientation, he or she is likely to help the client to do the same.

Problem management?

Before going further in this discussion of models for helping I should like to point out a difficulty. These theories and models are all directed to problem *management*. The nursing process is oriented towards problem *solving*. There is a big difference.

On the whole, nurses themselves are people who are problem solving oriented; that is, they see a nursing problem, identify it, and set out to resolve it. But counselling is different. In helping and counselling it is 'the individual, not the problem, (who) is the focus' (Rogers, 1942). In helping we are dealing with a person: a person with a problem.

As nursing becomes more holistic, it is argued that the whole person is now regarded, not just the part which is diseased; this is a step in the right direction. For most nurses, however, helping someone through counselling will still represent a complete change of emphasis.

The person presents a problem, but the problem is not the focus. If it is, then the process used is either advising or information giving. A problem has a *solution*; counselling works towards a *goal*. Counselling helps the *person*, and that means normally focusing on the person's *feelings* first of all, and then on the *meaning* of these feelings for the person.

The theories outlined are therefore called problem management because the person has to learn to manage a problem, not necessarily solve it. These aspects should become clearer as you read through the book, particularly when concentrating on the skills.

The stages of counselling

So that the theories of counselling may be seen to have practical possibilities, I shall describe here the stages, as outlined in Table 5.1, related to a specific example.

In a chapter entitled 'The myth and reality of interpersonal skills use in nursing', Cormack (1985) gives an example of interactions between a patient and his nurses. It is an anecdote of 'a young man who had to be hospitalised for medical treatment of an eye ailment'.

I shall first quote the story and then, with the help of the theories, imagine what the specific counselling interactions might have been like.

The impatience of the man during this, his first, hospitalisation, coupled with a natural shyness and feeling of inferiority, resulted in considerable anxiety and reluctance to stay for the duration of his treatment. When asked why he did stay and complete the treatment, he replied: 'It was because of the nurses. They made me feel welcome, they made me feel at home. After a while, they made me feel just like one of them. They made me want to stay and finish the treatment.'

Attending (Carkhuff) The story says that the patient was impatient, shy, feeling inferior, anxious and reluctant.

In attending to a patient or client you show that you are aware of these things but that they don't put you off. You stay with the person. You don't just say 'Good morning' as you pass the foot of his bed, but you go up to him. You give him your time, your attention, your energy, your knowledge. For the time being he is the only person that matters. When he has your attention then he also has his attention and has to concentrate on what is going on.

I imagine a conversation between this patient and a nurse could have started something like:

Patient: I don't think this treatment is helping me.
Nurse: What makes you think so?

Patient:	It's done nothing for me so far and I feel a fraud taking up a bed.
Nurse:	You are not a fraud, not a bit of it. Do I suspect a bit of impatience?
Patient:	A bit of it?! A great deal of it!
Nurse:	Do you think your eyes are worth waiting for a day or two to see how the treatment goes?
Patient:	All right, you win. When I look at it in that light, sure, they are worth waiting for.

This interaction simply shows that, by giving attention to the person, much can be achieved. If the nurse had simply replied 'Patience, man, patience!' to the original statement, he might have felt patronized and even more ready to leave, but the attention he got showed him that the nurse cared for him as a person, and that made him want to stay.

Define and identify the problem (Egan and Nelson-Jones) In any situation where you need to get somewhere it is best to know where you are starting from. In counselling, this means that the client has to describe the problem. This is often not easy at all.

> I don't know what's happening to me.
> I seem to have lost my grip of things.
> It's like being in a tunnel without any light at the end.

These and similar statements seem to be more common than

> I know exactly what I need (or want).

Very often, people find an 'obvious' problem as an entry to asking for help. This can be conscious and deliberate, wanting to see how the helper will respond before they expose their heart. It can also be a subconscious ploy so as *not* to look deeper.

> I've got such a headache today.
> If only this swallowing would improve, then I'd be perfectly all right.

Imagine that the example patient might have said

> I've never been in hospital before; I don't know how to fit into a routine.

These are all opening gambits and they may be the problem which a patient wants to come to terms with. This may well not be the 'real' problem. In order for the client to voice the real problem, and for the helper to hear it, a story needs to be told. This is often therapeutic in itself. Often a person may have been thinking over a problem, turning it round and round in his mind and never coming to a real conclusion. In *telling* it to someone, someone who hears and responds, a solution can present itself.

Sometimes there seem to be layers and layers of problems. One problem identified leads to half a dozen more to be discovered. At this stage the important element is to voice the problems, become aware of them and describe them.

Egan calls this 'the present scenario': that which is happening now. In order to make this stage objective, Egan asks 'What is the preferred scenario?' as a substage. Within this framework the preferred scenario is that the problem is recognized and attended to. The 'action' in this, the first stage, is to hold the problem present, and to agree to work on it.

An interaction between the example patient and nurse might therefore, starting with the same opening statement as before, be:

Patient: I don't think this treatment is helping me.
Nurse: What makes you think so?
Patient: It's done nothing for me so far and I feel a fraud taking up a bed.
Nurse: A fraud?
Patient: Well, yes, there's nothing really wrong with me that should keep me in hospital.
Nurse: I feel that you would rather not be here.
Patient: I can hardly stand it. Seeing all these other people around me gives me the shivers.
Nurse: You've never seen so many ill people before all together.
Patient: No, and I think it's going to be me next going blind.
Nurse: You sound as if you are really afraid of being blind.
Patient: I had never voiced it before, but yes, I know, that's what it's all about.
Nurse: Do you want to tell me about it?
Patient: I have always been too scared to face it but I can't avoid it now. Yes, do you have the time?

A real counselling conversation would probably have more interaction, but this shows the general direction of helping and counselling in this, the opening stage.
Responding to clients (Carkhuff) As well as setting a working frame for the counselling process, Carkhuff has

also established a four-point model of the essential features within that model:

1. Feeling
2. Reason
3. Meaning
4. Goal.

This makes it clear that if you want to help a person, then what matters first are the *feelings*. This is what most people have difficulty with. When they know how to deal with their feelings, then any problems can usually be dealt with because they are no longer a threat.

Identifying the feeling is not always easy. Because the person will tell a story, it will usually be the *facts* which are concentrated on. To respond appropriately to the person at this stage is therefore always to search for the feelings. This, simply put, is what responding empathically is about.

Feelings are never isolated. There is always a reason. And that reason constitutes the story. As you listen *to* the story and encourage its telling, you nevertheless listen *for* the feelings. What happened for this feeling to exist? What is happening now to the client as she or he is telling the story? What feelings does the story-telling engender?

In the story of the example patient (p. 44), the nurse picked up (empathy) that he is afraid of going blind. The feeling is fear, and by voicing this she was right into the main problem. She had responded in the best way, the only way, and the patient was then ready to tell her his story. He could begin to give the reason for his feelings. **Operationalize the problem(s)** (Nelson-Jones); **Personalize the experience** (Carkhuff). One of the most useful things a helper can do is to enable the client to see his problem in the context of life. A problem never appears out of the blue, and however much it may seem to be unrelated to other spheres of life, a few simple connections will usually give a totally different picture.

Once a problem has been identified and grasped, it needs to be made workable. Above all it needs to be made personal. The notion of self-responsibility has to come into the picture, and also the notion of what it all means.

They give me the shivers.
You make me so angry.
She shouldn't be allowed to do this to people.

These and similar statements are usually around at the beginning of a helping interaction. The client is behaving as a victim. In order now to tackle the problem, the client has to learn that the only people who are victims are those who allow themselves to be victims. Nobody *makes* him angry, but he *is* angry.

Nelson-Jones refers to skills deficits which have to be seen and identified. The problem can now be related to other areas of behaviour or attitudes. Patterns can be seen which put the problem into a wider context. Has this happened before? What did you do then?

The other powerful question here is about meaning. Does this problem have a meaning? Is it a defence mechanism? Is it a blind spot which protects something?

The 'problem' has now become only an identity-tag for the work that the person is doing. Because the person recognizes that what matters are his feelings and how they hinder or help him, he is no longer afraid and paralysed, but able to function more fully.

Imagine what the example patient might be telling the nurse:

Patient: Do you have time to listen?
Nurse: I am all ears.
Patient: Well, where to begin? There was this boy at school ...
            My grandmother was almost blind for years ... She
            couldn't really cope, but she refused help ... She
            impressed me both by her independence and by the way
            her clothes were always stained with food.
Nurse: Having an eye problem now makes you relate to her and
            you think one day you will be stubborn and off-putting
            to others by wearing food-stained clothes?
Patient: You guessed!
Nurse: Have you ever been in such a situation?
Patient: Well, you could say I am now; I don't fit in here, and I
            wanted to go home, and I can't see enough with this
            treatment, so I may spill tea or toothpaste down my front.
Nurse: I sense that you are afraid of losing control, and also of
            having to conform.
Patient: I am afraid of getting old, of being ill, and not having
            achieved anything in my life.

The underlying questions are: what is happening to this

person? what is the meaning of the fear of blindness?

The interaction would no doubt go on for a while but, sooner or later, in order to make this helping relevant, the counsellor has to point to a goal.

Goal development (Egan); **Initiating action** (Carkhuff); **Setting goals** (Nelson-Jones) Having become aware of the problem and then paid attention to it, the next step is one of choice: what to do with it? Egan calls this the stage of getting out of the morass.

Galbraith (1979) believes that one of the reasons why poor people remain poor is that they accept themselves as poor and do not even imagine themselves as not poor. Egan thinks that many clients remain in their morass because they don't imagine, and are not helped to imagine, a future different from the present one. He believes that 'the most underused resource in clients is imagination'. The question is: 'What would it be like if your world were just a little better?'. Most people would like their world to be a lot better, but by trying to manage too much they may not be able to manage at all. This is the reason for asking for a world a *little* better: a little better at each point in the process.

Carkhuff, with his emphasis on development and growing, also sees developing goals as the aim of the helping process.

Nelson-Jones writes of choosing and negotiating treatment interventions.

This is the stage where the counsellor's skills become particularly evident. It is too easy to slip into the advising mode:

If I were you I would . . . .
What you need to do is . . . .

This simply shows up *your* goals, not those of the client. This is something that must be kept firmly in mind, otherwise the whole process is ruined. Carkhuff is adamant that helping is always 'for better or for worse', but never for neutral. It is for better or for worse here mainly because of the helper's skills (LaMonica et al, 1976).

It is often a necessary step at this stage to help the patient or client to get deeply in touch with the 'morass'. This is the present scenario of Egan's first substage at this, his stage 2. You can only move forward when you know where you are starting from. This morass is usually so uncomfortable that a client would give anything to be rid of it. Nevertheless, without having owned it, recognized responsibility for it, and thuse chosen to move forward, there is never going to be a clear goal.

The essence of this stage is therefore 'the preferred scenario'. Egan calls this 'futuring'. The client looks forward, and commits himself to the future. To help the client achieve this, the helper has to do a fair amount of challenging, interpreting and confronting, and this can prove painful. The basis of the helper's right to challenge is support. She needs to encourage and respect the client, and must also believe in her client's ability to cope and manage.

Look at the example patient again, and imagine in your own mind how this goal-setting might be achieved. In my own words, they may be saying something like this to each other, picking the conversation up from p. 48:

Patient: I am afraid of getting old, of being ill, and not having achieved anything in my life.

Nurse: There is another fear now, that of getting old. And there is a fear of not using your life fully.

Patient: The fear of getting old and being ill is quite overpowering.

Nurse: Do you equate being old and being ill?

Patient: To an extent, yes.

Nurse: You are ill now, but you are not old.

Patient: I hadn't thought of it that way. Perhaps that's why I am impatient now, because I am not old, but I feel old and helpless with this illness.

Nurse: You are touching on more and more aspects of yourself. Which do you think is the one which matters most at this moment?

Patient: Well – right now, I think, being impatient.

Nurse: What would your world look like if you were less impatient?

Patient: I would accept that I am ill and need this treatment.

Nurse: It sounds quite easy. Is it?

Patient: Yes and no. You are helping me to see that it could be less difficult than I thought.

Nurse: How are you going to be less impatient? Or should I say, how are you going to be more patient?

Patient: Saying it like this makes it possible to tackle it. Being more patient – yes, that's what it is. That might also put the other issues and fears into a more manageable perspective.

Again, this is not how a 'real' conversation would go. There would probably be many more interactions in between. Perhaps also some pauses, questions, 'don't know's and encouraging 'um's and a good deal of body language which can be revealing of a person's feelings. However, the general trend can be seen. The patient is gradually working towards owning the feelings, taking responsibility for them, moving forward by imagining 'a better tomorrow', and finally taking action in doing something to get out of the morass on to more comfortable and sure ground.

Intervene (Nelson-Jones) Perhaps Egan and Carkhuff trust their clients enough, after setting goals, to go and carry them out. This is a very positive approach and would demonstrate that there is now the possibility for the client *to* act. But Nelson-Jones has a point in continuing his model into actually 'doing'.

However well goals are set and perhaps tried out, most people meet some difficulty. The person who has learnt to be more assertive and now sets forth to *be* assertive will still find that occasionally it is difficult, and makes a mistake. That is then precisely the moment when the client needs support and perhaps more help in re-examining the goals and re-negotiating interventions. Therefore, to spell out again how the goal is put into practice is a good and always helpful point.

Patient: Being more patient – yes, that's what it is.
Nurse: That's a very good point. How are you going to do it?
Patient: Telling myself to be patient.
Nurse: It sounds as if this is just a bit too easy – as if you always tell yourself to be patient
Patient: (astonished) You are reading me like a book! Yes, I often tell myself to be patient, and – coming to think of it, I usually end up being more impatient than before.
Nurse: So how are you going to be patient now?
Patient: I am going to stay here and I'm going to see the treatment through. And I'm not going to moan but I'm going to be positive about it because you helped me see the point of it all. Can I help *you* with anything around the ward?

Exit (Nelson-Jones) A good helping relationship has a good beginning, middle and end. Each aspect is important. Sadly, the end, or exit, is often a neglected area.

The interaction which I have traced through this chapter is a one-off, short episode. There will be many of these in every nurse's work; but there will also be the long-term relationships.

The example I used concentrated first on fear, and then became more immediate by focusing on impatience. Fear is something so common that it underlies many of our behaviours and attitudes. But the other, and just as strong, element in most people's lives is loss. Being ill is then another loss. Being helped through counselling is a restoration, but having that help terminated or withdrawn may bring the whole problem back again and even make it worse. The ending of a relationship is therefore crucial, and may need to be carefully prepared.

But Nelson-Jones also views this point of the helping model as an evaluation. A review is taking place and the learning achieved can be consolidated. This can be particularly helpful. Few people remember exactly what their starting point was and how they have changed, and what has changed. To be able to do such a review with a client can prove to be quite invaluable, and is always encouraging.

Imagine the example patient one more time:

Patient: I'm going to stay here . . . Can I help you with anything around the ward?

Nurse: By staying you are actually helping yourself and me too – we are only two sides of one coin! By helping me – that's great, you show that you are serious about what we just discussed. Can you sit with P. for a while, he feels a bit lonely?

Patient: You mean doing to him what you just did to me?

Nurse: Sort of, yes!

Patient: I'm not a counsellor.

Nurse: You don't have to be, but he said something about the day being long this morning.

Patient: I get the point: patience!

Nurse: I'm around if you need help.

This extract shows a form of exiting, and also how self-help skills can be consolidated. The nurse encourages him to use these straight away, and practising is the best way to prove that what you preach is valid.

Making this, the last stage in the helping relationship, right is important for the client as well as for the helper. A relationship left open, unfinished, perhaps painful, is always difficult. It is not always possible to leave your client on a 'high', but to leave him floundering may be destructive. Leaving clients quietly crying may be all right in some circumstances; leaving them in a rage may not. But simply plastering over cracks may not be all right either. A relationship is only really ended when the feelings of both parties are OK, and for that to happen, you have to be responsible for *your* feelings.

The non-linear model

The models just presented move in a linear way from A to B to C. The model is neat: but life isn't!

Egan is quite clear in his writings that nothing is a law: everything is organic. What matters is that counselling helps the client in whichever form it is applied.

There are not only 'high-level counsellors', there are also 'high-level clients'. They may come to you with an awareness of their problems which shows that they have gone backwards and forwards through all the stages. For one reason or another, they now need or want help from you. You may need to make a quick judgement and decide at what stage the client is. You may also need to be very flexible and be as empathic as possible with your responses without finding a label or a stage. All models are here to help *you*, not to fit the client into a role. It is perhaps significant that Egan, who developed a clear model, has symbolized it by two circles; his model is particularly non-linear.

The four questions

Over many years of counselling practice, inside and outside nursing, I have developed my own guidelines which I should like to present.

I have always used some model to help me keep to a direction in counselling. Without some signposts I find that I can go round and round the problem without achieving anything. But if a model is too long, or too complicated, it is not much use to me either, because it becomes a question of following the model, and not the person. When I discovered the simple four-word model of Carkhuff (p. 47) I felt I could use it, but still in a way be free to be myself. I did not have to think of stages any more, but I felt a little concerned that this model did not finish clearly enough. Simply leaving a 'goal' is like a New Year's resolution: it is not based on something concrete, spelled out and committed to.

The four questions which I now use constantly as my guidelines for helping and counselling are loosely based on that model.

1. *What is happening*? What is going on here? What is the person saying or not saying? What is going on between

us (client and helper)? What am I hearing? What am I not hearing?

2. *What is the meaning of it?* What significance does the problem have in your (the client's) life? What memories does it bring up? What patterns does it show? What purpose is there in the problem; in the help sought?

3. *What is your goal?* What aim do you have now? What is changing as you talk about your problem and about yourself?

4. *How are you going to do it?* How are you going to commit yourself to the new vision? What *practical* steps are you going to take to change?

These four questions evolved and emerged from other people's writings, from what I heard myself say to clients, from management strategies I met, and perhaps even from my unconscious, because one morning they seemed just to be there, perfectly obvious.

Some of the advantages of having a model in the form of questions are:

a) It keeps the focus on the client. By asking the client these specific questions it helps you to concentrate on the client, not on your own need to keep to a model.

b) It makes the client work. You are less likely to propose your own solutions, but help the client to find his or her goals.

c) They are open questions. They are models to the use of other open questions in the process.

d) They can also apply to your own evaluation of a session, or process.

e) They are not exclusive, but can be asked differently in different circumstances.

This is perhaps what should happen to any model: use it, discard it, try something else. In the end what matters is that you are confident with your skills and that you help in the way which is best and unique for you. Then you are a *person* helping another *person*.

There are of course many other models available for helping and counselling such as Gestalt (Perls, 1973), Neuro-linguistic programming (Bandler, 1985), Psycho-drama (Goldman and Morrison, 1984), Transactional analysis (Berne, 1964; Harris, 1973), Psychosynthesis

(Ferrucci, 1982), Client-centred therapy (Rogers, 1951), Reality therapy (Glasser, 1965), Behavioural counselling (Krumboltz and Thorenson, 1969).

6 Learning counselling

Are you a counsellor?

It has sometimes been argued that if the helper is empathic enough, nothing else is needed. He or she is then an entirely eclectic (not belonging to any recognized 'school' or system) worker, freely using various sources for helping. Other people have argued that if you keep to a well-structured theory or model, that is enough, because both helper and client know the way. Yet others have thought that by having a wide range of skills available, helping happens because the helper *is* so skilled.

There is some truth in each of these approaches. Most people however, are neither totally empathic, totally theoretical, or totally skilled to work only in one mode. Most people find that they need a mix of empathy, theory and skills.

Another assumption sometimes made is that counsellors are born, not made. Could it be that people who don't want to be counsellors think that?

I believe that the skills play a large part in counselling. Just as a nurse has to acquire the skill of giving an injection, so she or he can also acquire the skills of counselling. True, one is a motor skill and the other is a communication skill; but both are *skills* which, according to the *Oxford English Dictionary*, are 'a practised ability, dexterity, facility in doing something'. While skills *can* be learnt, not everybody learns them to the same degree. Nor is this necessary. We cannot all be experts in everything. It matters less that you have a wide range of skills than that you use the skills you have.

Reading about counselling in a book can make it seem remarkably easy. It is when you actually practise it that everything goes wrong. It is then too easy to blame the book, or the process or the client, and give up. Therefore I should like to warn you: expect difficulties! Nothing is easy; everything has to be practised. As you practise, you will get confidence, and as your confidence grows, so your expertise grows. But I would also say, trust the skills you already have, and use them. Anything that you learn is extra.

Learning counselling skills

All forms of helping and counselling are interpersonal; they happen between and among people. Essentially, therefore, learning counselling is also best done interpersonally, between and among people. Ideally, counselling is learnt in a group and over a period of time, in the company of a person competent to facilitate the learning.

But such learning needs to be assimilated. That is where books have their place. At home, away from the actual situation, it is possible to 'read, learn, mark and inwardly digest' what has gone on in real life. That is when you learn on your own.

'Which is the best book to read to learn more about counselling?' is a question sometimes asked but impossible to answer. Some books are more basic, others more theoretical. Some books stress one aspect, others some different area. They all contain invaluable insights. Most of them speak out of the experience of the writer, and that is inevitably different from your own, but hopefully you can relate to it. When you can do that, reading a book becomes like a counselling relationship: you attend to what you read, you respond to it with the occasional 'ah!' and you are challenged by it.

One important form of learning counselling is learning how to listen. Many people think they are good listeners, and that may be true. But I believe that we can never listen well enough and constantly need to learn to listen more, and better, and have our listening capacities challenged. A few listening exercises which you can do on your own or with a colleague are described below.

Learning listening

Listening is the central skill and act of counselling. To be able to listen, you need to be silent. Learning on your own how to listen is not easy, as listening is done only in relation to someone, or something. When you learn to listen you will probably be surprised to find that you hear 'sounds' which were there, but which you never heard.

Listening is first of all a physical activity. At the level of the ear, the physical organ of hearing, you hear, you perceive and notice. This level of awareness is also necessary in helping, as it brings the body and the mind together.

In a quiet place sound all the vowels, A E I O U, one after the other, and slowly. Listen to the echo. Listen also to the sounds they make within you.

Sit quietly for five minutes and consciously listen to all the sounds you hear. Make a note of what these are.

Listen to some music and with your body express what the sounds convey to you at that moment.

Close your eyes and 'listen' to what your face says to you: the forehead, the eyebrows, the eyes, the nose, the cheeks, the lips, the jaw. Be aware of these parts of you. Follow up, in whatever way seems appropriate, what each reveals to you.

At your next meal follow a piece of bread, a spoonful of custard, or other food into your mouth, through the oesophagus, stomach and intestine. Notice where it stops of its own accord, and what it does there. Do this several times and notice when your attention lapses.

Look at a photograph of someone. Then close your eyes and remember that person. Remember as many details as possible. Then open your eyes and compare your memory with the photograph.

Put yourself into the position most related to the present mood. Change the position as the mood changes.

Many people find that they have blind spots and mental blockages somewhere along the line. Sometimes an exercise to get in touch with the body will reveal a physical blockage, real or perceived, which can help you to understand any mental blockage better. You can do these exercises for yourself, and help teach your clients to do them too, thus increasing their understanding of themselves.

One way of learning to listen to what is actually said, the words spoken, is to write out a conversation. Take any conversation you had with family, friends, or at work. As soon as possible after the event try to write down as accurately as possible how the conversation went. Notice where you can't remember what was said; where you don't remember what you said or what the other person said.

You will probably have forgotten some parts of the conversation, or remember the last part better than the middle part. This is perfectly normal. When you think that you have to remember such a conversation you will pay much more careful attention to the words, but in doing so you may be less aware of yourself and the other person.

A more advanced way of learning to listen to others is by the use of a tape recorder. But first of all a word of warning. When using a tape recorder with patients, you must be sure they are aware of being taped and you must gain their consent to it. Not to do so infringes their right to confidentiality. If a friend or member of the family is taped, a judgement would have to be made as to whether personal rights or spontaneity are more important. Any use of recording equipment inhibits a person, including yourself, at least to begin with.

If possible, tape a conversation. Start with a short, five-minute interaction. Stop the tape. Then try to remember what was said, and write the conversation down. Then listen to the tape, and compare what was said and what you have written. By going over the tape and the written piece a few times, you may become aware of the areas which you either forgot or distorted in your writing. Pay attention to such distortions, and notice any reasons for this.

An audio tape has the disadvantage of not conveying gestures and movements. If a video tape is available, these aspects are included. If possible, ensure that both helper and client are monitored. If this is not possible, a tape of any conversation on film can be used. Watch it once. Write out what you remember, and then watch it again, and compare the film with your written records.

These exercises will never replace the real situations and the learning which goes on there, but they can sharpen your listening acuity.

Listening exercises can be learnt on your own, but all helping skills are ideally learnt in groups. Learning together in groups is not only fun, but also safe when well done. Remember: you are not in a real-life situation.

You can try out different approaches, and you get feedback on your performance, which is probably the single biggest advantage of learning in groups.

Here are two exercises for learning listening which can be done in groups of three people:

1. Learner 1 talks for two minutes, telling Learner 2 about her present work. Learner 2 then talks to Learner 3, telling her what Learner 1 does, introducing her, so to speak.

    This can be done in different ways. It need not only be about work; a topic of interest or an item from the day's news can be used in this way.

    Every learner should take a turn at being 1, 2 and 3. Learner 1 then tells Learner 3 if Learner 2 has (a) repeated well what Learner 1 said; (b) omitted anything; (c) told the story in the right sequence

    The next exercise may be more difficult:

2. Two of the three people talk normally on a subject in which the third person is interested or experienced but the third person stays silent. She then tells the two speakers what she experienced during this exercise: frustration, jealousy, curiosity, ambiguity.

    This exercise helps you to learn not to criticize others, not to put forward your own opinions when they have not been called for.

    In any group exercise, feedback is always as important as the exercise itself. Only when you hear what you have done well, or less well, do you have guidelines and clarity for improvement. The most important person to give feedback is always the speaker. Self-evaluation is more valuable than anything else; in real life you have only yourself to measure against. Therefore it is also essential to learn in groups.

Learning about feelings

It is very easy to make assumptions. We imagine that other people think and act like we do; or if they don't, that they should.

You may be saying you are feeling well, although you have just spilled your coffee, have premenstrual tension and are dreading going to a particular patient. Your neighbour may, under the same circumstances, say that she is feeling dreadful.

Rather than assume, particularly with feelings, it is important to learn to discern the client's feelings. Some feelings are strong, some weak. Some are obvious and some are hidden. Some feelings we can describe very well; others are ambiguous, unclear or mixed.

Learning about counselling is often learning about feelings. Listen to how feelings

a) Are expressed.
b) Are hidden.
c) Are wanting to be expressed.
d) Are about something, and what that is.
e) Are implying a meaning.
f) Are wanting to create meaning.
g) Are about movement.

Listen to your own feelings, and take them seriously. Then you will be hearing more empathically what your client's feelings are.

Learning other skills

Many of the skills detailed in the next few chapters can also be learnt on your own. Here are some ideas for doing this.

a) The next time you have a telephone conversation, take a mirror and watch yourself. Notice your body language: your smiles, the way you move your lips, your jaw, your shoulders. If you can sit in front of a full-length mirror, then you can watch your whole body. Look at yourself as if you were the recipient of these expressions. Do you like what you see? Does anything put you off? How 'helpful' are your eyes, your posture? Give yourself a mark for *attending* to the other person.

b) If you want to learn one specific skill, say clarifying, give yourself a day for it. Notice every time when you are clarifying something in a conversation. Notice when you are not doing it. How well do you do it? What difficulty do you have with it? You could also ask individual friends or colleagues to help you with it. Tell them that that is what you particularly want to learn, and ask them to give you feedback every time they have been aware that you are clarifying something. This is possible with every skill, although you may find it easier with some than with others.

There are possibilities for challenging yourself and your views about helping and counselling. Try the following:

c) Write down in the form of a letter to a close friend: What helping and/or counselling means to you.

What your reason is for wanting to counsel others.
What you get out of counselling.

d)   Write out a character description of yourself:
     How do you see yourself?
     How do you think others see you?

These and other exercises which you can devise for
yourself help you to become aware of yourself as a person
and as a helper. Such exercises are not ends in themselves.
They point to the wider picture: it is out of the
understanding of yourself that you can understand others
and help them to understand themselves.

Nurse (1980) says:

There is no doubt that any type of caring relationship
makes demands on both parties and the greater the
awareness and perception the counsellor has (not
necessarily comparable with the number of years she
has lived!) the greater the contribution she can make to
others. This experience is by no means confined to that
which is outward – more important is the inward
experience which she has gained from self-knowledge
and self-realisation.

Self-knowledge and self-evaluatoin are essential skills
in helping. Both evolve out of constant learning and
working at improving skills.

7 Counselling skills: attending

Attending

You have probably said, and had said to you, 'You're not listening to what I'm saying'. However much you protest, and can repeat every word the accuser said, the effect remains. People don't want words repeated; they want the person to be 'all there'.

Attending is so simple, and often also so difficult, that it is coming to be seen more and more as a basic and important skill of helping, worthy of a good deal of research (Egan, 1986). Carkhuff makes it the starting point of his model for helping (see Table 5.1).

Attending means that you orient yourself towards the client. You are with this person in body, mind and spirit, imparting the sense that your client is the only person that matters at the moment. You turn off your bleep or telephone. You ensure, as far as possible, that you are sitting at the same height and in chairs of similar construction, that the room is comfortably warm and the lighting appropriate. If you have a drink, you both use similar cups.

Enviroment

These basics are the ideal, even the theoretical. We all know that much counselling and helping takes place during bed-bathing and tub-bathing, in linen cupboards, on the doorstep and in noisy dining rooms. But given the chance, often with a minimum of effort, these conditions can be improved. When you are sensitive to the needs of others, they may not even notice that you are helping them in this way.

When you have a chance, notice the effect created when you sit and swivel in your comfortable office armchair, while your client sits in a moulded fibreglass chair; or when your patient is lying down in bed and you sit on the edge; or there is a table between you. Clutching the shoulders of someone bursting into tears then becomes quite a performance.

Most of all though, what matters is that *you are there*. You are with that person; not with the client you have just left, your evening guests, or what you are about to tell the boss. When you can be with each of these in their own time you will be more effective there and then, and also save yourself a good deal of mental energy.

Culture and language

When you attend a patient, you enter that person's world. That may be a very different world from your own. In a sense it is true that feelings of love and hate are the same the world over, but how they are expressed are not. When people are ill, their basic patterns and instincts tend to become more important because they are 'in the blood'. Different customs concerning food and hygiene have become increasingly familiar and acknowledged, but some religious practices may not yet be so widely understood.

Perry (1988) makes the point that a helping intervention may be interpreted as 'Babylon' by a Rastafarian, and thus as evidence of the oppression of his people. An Asian person may not want to take part in any treatment, including counselling, outside a setting where the whole family is involved; this may apply particularly to women. In that setting, concepts of 'self-determination' and 'self-responsibility' are irrelevant because the culture does not value personal autonomy.

One patient may say that he can only be washed at a time when the evil spirits are not around; another converses with the spirits. When the culture and language of a particular patient are not our own, we are often quick to dismiss unfamiliar practices and to impose our own routines and standards. But this diminishes the person. Attending – really hearing what the person says – may at times mean a trip to a library to read more about a particular culture; or it may mean learning to adapt our language to that of the client.

Even in Britain there is a big difference between the culture of North and South. How much greater is the problem when there are also differences of race and language. Listening to another person involves so much.

Body language

The body language of both people in an interaction is important. Egan has described the helper's physical attending with the acronym SOLER:

Squarely: Face the client **S**quarely. This can be meant both physically (sitting opposite) and metaphorically (conveying the message 'I am with you').

Open: Adopt an **O**pen posture. Crossed arms and legs can be signs of closing off. Your posture should convey 'I am open to you'.

Lean: It is possible to **L**ean towards the other. Leaning towards the other person can be seen as 'I am interested in you'.

Eye: Maintain **E**ye contact. This is a comfortable contact, not a staring. It is a way of saying 'I am with you; I want to hear what you have to say'.

Relaxed: Try to be **R**elaxed. Nervousness and fidgeting are easily transmitted. This can make an unsure patient even more uncomfortable. When you are relaxed, the client can also relax.

None of this is a rule, rather a reminder of aspects of helping which, when you are yourself, you do anyway.

Paying attention to the client's body language is the other side of the coin. Notice his posture, facial expression, breathing, nervousness, eye contact. Most nurses are very good at observation; you can make use of these aspects for your helping. The sense of *sight* can be used very effectively and you can feed this back to a patient.

When you said that you uncrossed your arms. Is it a relief to have said it?
A frown came across your forehead just then – is this something which is troubling you?
Your face brightened up as you said that.
That was a deep sigh – what happened there?

The sense of *hearing* is in the listening. You listen not only to the words, but also to the tone of the words and their speed. Does the client have a dry mouth? Does speech come easily? Does your client use plain speech or metaphors? Paying attention to what is said and how it is said can give you insights which are useful to you, and which the client gives away, probably without being aware of it; you get the insight 'for free'.

You can also make use of *smell*. You can gain a lot of information from the way both men and women use smells and scents to enhance their image, and which part of that image they enhance or neglect. A client who is very depressed is less likely to use scent and dress well.

A counselling relationship, however, may be a turning point, and if you notice a change in appearance, comment on it and encourage it.

On many occasions the request 'come and smell my lovely roses' has been the opening a patient was looking for to talk to a nurse. You should never underestimate such an invitation.

You may not often be called upon to use the sense of *taste*, but you could be in situations when patients offer you sweets, or a cup of tea, or some other titbit to eat. This can be an important token of sharing.

Touch, the last sense, plays an important part in helping. When you get nearer to people emotionally, you also get nearer physically. As a nurse you often have close physical contact with many people, but little emotional contact. But it is not a reciprocal contact: nurses touch patients, but by and large patients don't touch nurses.

Some people who are disturbed and frightened want very close contact; others want to be left alone. When you can read the body language of such people you will probably help in the most appropriate way.

It is perhaps the sense of touch which is the most difficult and also the most pertinent of the senses in helping. Without words you can convey deep caring with an arm around a shoulder. Or you can cradle a person like a child while he or she cries and lets go of tension and pent-up emotions. At such moments you overstep any norms of touching, and barriers of 'right' conduct are forgotten. When you help someone, you do so essentially as another human being, and this is nowhere more clearly demonstrated than in the act of touching and being touched. The language of the body is used not only to reveal aspects of the client's life to you, but you also use it to convey to the client that you are 'with' and 'for' that person.

Giving space

With understanding and empathy you move into the other's world; you invade his territory, so to speak. This is the territory of feelings, behaviours and experiences.

> Man's use of space has a bearing on his ability to relate to other people, to sense them as being close or far away. (Fast, 1971)

Nurses are in a very privileged position from which they invade people's territory all day and every day. They wash people, clean their teeth for them, give them enemas, deliver their babies, change their colostomy bags. Much of this is done to people who are almost, or completely, naked. They are going much closer than even a close family member might go in physical contact. It should not be astonishing, then, that such people also let you into their intimate personal space, or, alternatively, that they resent this and drive you out.

This territory of feelings, experiences and meaning is often like a moor, or a wood. There is a lot of growth on the ground. There are also unnoticed stones, holes, roots, perhaps caves and ravines. These things need to be experienced and noticed. Most of this is done by the client telling you about all this, telling you his story.

> By patiently listening to the distraught man, by being present for him, we give him space to think and to feel. Perhaps, instead of speaking of space and time, it would be truer to say that the patient man gives the other room to live; he enlarges the other's living room. (Mayeroff, 1972)

People need to roam about in their thoughts, go down memory lane and build castles in the air; they need permission to talk and explore the inner country; they may need little more than the occasional word of encouragement; or they may need you as a companion in this exploration.

By being aware of the need for space you give the client something vital. You give him, or help him to give himself, his own self. When you are invited by a client into his space, then you are in the privileged position of helper.

Depending upon your own sense of space, you may need to practise going in and out of other people's space, and how you use your own space.

Perhaps with a friend, explore the space around you. How much space do you need? Ask your friend to act as if she were ill: how much space does she want or need? If she is happy, thoughtful, distraught, or waiting for the result of a test – practise on each other how your space influences you.

Timing and pacing

The time you have available for help will greatly influence the process of helping itself. When there is pressure, you can do as much work in ten minutes as in one hour and ten minutes. Helping a person with a speech impairment will always take longer than helping a person who can talk normally.

Some clients are themselves quick people: others are slow. Some helpers are more energetic than others. A really deep-seated, painful problem cannot be exposed or explained quickly. On the other hand, some problems are very pressing. Will a patient accept a certain treatment? If not, what are his reasons and his resources for otherwise coping? The parents of a handicapped baby may have to decide within hours or days what they think is the best course of action in a given set of circumstances. Other patients may not have to make a decision for some time.

It may be appropriate not only to push patients and relatives in a helping situation, but also to slow them down. A quick decision may be a panic decision, and helpers may have to be firm and look at certain unclear or reluctant areas quite firmly.

Some people need far more time with one aspect than with another. It may be unrealistic to think that because yesterday a patient or relative needed twenty minutes of time, today he will need the same amount of time for a new aspect which may have arisen.

When you are 'with' the person, attending to your client fully, you will be aware of his or her time needs. To have some boundaries is often helpful (see p. 117), but boundaries are only valid when they can be broken.

You might like to think how you use your time in helping. What does your pressure of time convey to the client? It is a truism that half the world has too little time and the other half has too much. Fitting these two opposites together in helping is often like juggling. It is also an act of judgement to know whose time is more valuable; who has less of it?

Staying open   Staying open in helping means accepting, giving permission and listening. It also means that, as a helper, you go where the client wants to go. You follow your client's agenda, not yours; although as part of the counselling process you may bring a client to face a difficult issue by staying closely on that subject.

Patient: I believe there is something better than this at the end of it all, but I don't want to go yet. (Patient suppresses a tear.)

> *Nurse*: You said just now that crying is a safety valve for you, and I am sure you are using it as just that.
> *Patient*: That's it (Patient sniffs.)
> *Nurse*: You feel like crying?
> *Patient*: That's it, you're right.
> *Nurse*: I mean, do you want to cry now?
> *Patient*: A bit. But it doesn't do any harm. (Patient cries, then laughs, and cries again.)

By staying open to what is happening, you are not judging a person. You remain non-directive. You are open and ready to go with the client. Only by staying open will you be able to offer a person the safety to go on talking, particularly if it is painful. So often, patients come to the brink of talking about something important, delicate or painful, and then stop. 'I mustn't worry you. You might think me morbid.' To say something like 'You are not worrying me. Tell me about it' will give that permission, and may be the turning point for a person in mental distress.

In a way, the skill of staying open sums up all the skills of attending. None of these skills are easy, because they demand that you are all 'there'. By staying open you risk being hurt, becoming involved, getting tired, being exploited and used. But it is only by staying open that you can come close to another person and see change happen. The deep satisfaction in helping is that you can often see such changes and realize that, without your openness and your own vulnerability, this might not have come about, at least not in the same way.

The next three sections are not so much about practical skills of attending as aspects of empathy at this level of helping.

Being non-judgemental

'The highest expression of empathy is accepting and (being) non-judgemental' (Rogers, 1980). Rogers goes on to tell the story of a psychologist who was researching people's visual and perceptual history, including difficulties with seeing and reading. He simply listened to the subjects with interest and so gathered his data. To his surprise a number of them came back to thank him for his help. In his opinion he had given them no help at all. It made him 'recognize that interested non-evaluative listening is a potent therapeutic force'.

Martin (1977) makes a similar point:

> She sat and talked and talked. After about 45 minutes she looked at her watch and reached for her shopping bag.
> 'Well, Doctor, I really must be going, but thank you once again for all the advice – I don't know what I'd do without it.'
> For three-quarters of an hour I'd listened to the good lady *without saying a single word* – except 'good morning' of course. What is more, it had been just the same each time we'd met over the preceding three months.

You wouldn't survive in life without making judgements. As a nurse you have to make many judgements every day.

The next time you admit a new patient, be aware how many judgements you will have formed before you have been together for five minutes. The name, the age, the diagnosis, the handshake, the patient's clothes: these are all ways in which a person is 'revealed'. But are you correct?

It is not so long since nurses were refusing to treat patients with human immunodeficiency virus (HIV). Nurses made a judgement about these patients, and they judged negatively.

If you can set aside the patient's name, accent, colour of hair and diagnosis . . .

If you can set aside his need for three sugars in his coffee, his dislike of baths and his habit of smacking his thigh . . .

If you can set aside her use of your least favourite perfume, her constant late arrival, her silly nickname for her husband . . .

If you can hear what he says as being *his* story and his truth . . .

If you can believe what he says, despite what you think . . .

If you can show respect without thinking of how this affects you . . .

If you can do all this, then you are meeting a *person*, not a uniform, a preconceived idea, or a diagnosis.

> This patient declared one morning that she needed to be moved to the single room so that she could die in peace. She was ill, but she was not considered to be on the verge of death. Something in her voice took me

aback. I could not argue with her. I had a single room available, and I moved her, somehow waiting to be proved wrong. She telephoned all her relatives, one after the other, to come to her bedside. She asked her nephew to close her bank account and to help her make her will. When all this was done, she simply laid down again and died.

You will probably have your own story about the importance of being non-judgemental. If not, think of your patients, and be aware when you were last judgemental and how much you could help them; and when you were non-judgemental, and the help you were able to give then.

Encouraging

Anything unexpected, particularly illness and loss, usually leads to some loss of confidence.

I was managing alright, now I just can't.
I thought I was doing so well, until this happened.

Such loss may be temporary, or it may only be the beginning of a downward slide into incompetence. One way of compensating is by becoming aggressive. Another way is to abandon oneself to the 'sick' role, or to revert to childlike behaviour (see p. 23). Most people are not very self-assured to begin with, and a blow of any kind will render them paralysed.

A blocked and paralysed person cannot, however, move forward and change anything. A person who has no self-trust cannot imagine that life could be different.

The first step in any kind of helping is usually an awareness exercise. For whatever reason, someone who needs help is like a china doll. It was a beautiful doll, but something or someone smashed it up. It is lying in pieces on the floor. Parts of it are perfectly recognizable. But it cannot put itself together again on its own.

A glued-together doll will always be fragile and probably ugly. But a shattered person who is helped to come together again is much stronger for the experience. Nevertheless, some people do remain broken, scarred and in pieces. For whatever reason, they have chosen that path. People can be 'mended'; that is, they can have operations to correct diseased parts, and they can have medications to put some other aspect of the body right again. But they remain 'dolls'. They are not fully alive because the purpose for being ill does not exist any more.

Such people can only be approached with compassion, not with a zeal to change them. Real empathy accepts a person, and in that very acceptance may lie the seed for change.

The person who is able and willing to allow you to help her or him to gather the pieces together has already taken a vital first step. As a helper it is important (to continue with the metaphor) to point out and look at the pieces which are still intact, or the large bits which are clearly visible. Make sure that the client sees them too. When your individual clients see hope, strengthen it. When they tell you that they are feeling better today, be pleased with them.

Before any helping or actual counselling, and therefore changing, can be done, what is already there has to be seen and strengthened. Not only does what a client sees and tells you need to be encouraged; the whole person needs to be encouraged.

Patient: I feel I am not a good mother to my children any more.
Nurse: It's difficult at the moment. But you have been a good mother in the past, and after this you will be one again.
Patient: Do you really think that?
Nurse: Absolutely, I have no doubt.

Patient: I could do it, but not very well.
Nurse: You did it much better than I normally manage it.

Patient: I don't know if I have the guts now to stand up to him.
Nurse: It will be difficult, I agree. But just a few moments ago I notice you being quietly assertive getting your meal. What you could do there you can do with him too.

People who have been damaged are generally aware of the damage; in this way they are in touch with negativity, darkness and helplessness. By encouragement, you are gradually putting before them a different mode of being and behaving and, out of this, change can happen.

Empowering

Counselling is goal-oriented. It is a form of helping by which eventually the client can live more resourcefully and satisfyingly. This means that he or she will have acquired some self-help skills. Empowering is about fostering these skills, and making the client independent and ceasing to rely on others.

It has been said that preparation for discharge starts when a patient is admitted. In the same way, in order for the client to have a good 'exit' (Nelson-Jones) from a counselling relationship, the territory has to be prepared right from the start.

Many clients put counsellors in the position of 'saviour': they expect to be pulled out of the morass by some superforce or super-person; many so-called counsellors fall into the trap and 'save' others. The fact is that we can never save others; we can only point out to clients the tools and methods of how to help themselves out of the morass.

Egan (1986) likes to refer to helpers as consultants, thus making it clear that they use the client's own resources rather than being the 'more knowing' party of the two. The client who wants and needs to be helped is therefore first helped to see what are the strengths, resources and means already there. The helper is then not that saviour or rescuer, but a collaborator for change.

This can often sound quite hard for patients to take.

Patient: I thought you were going to help me.
Nurse: I will, and I can do that to the extent that you are helping yourself.

Listening

The wise old owl sat in an oak
The more he saw the less he spoke
The less he spoke the more he heard
Why can't we all be like that bird?

I listen, hopefully in such a way that the person of my concern will hear, from deep within, the decisions which he or she has to make and act upon.
(Kirkpatrick, 1985)

Listening is the beginning and end of helping, and also its middle. The first of the four questions (What is happening?) is the question of and for listening.

Listening is something active. You are not only sitting and letting your ears do the work. Active listening means listening to both the verbal and non-verbal messages of those who come to you for help. In a way, you have to listen with all your senses, and on the level of the senses. Ways of sitting, dressing, smelling, looking, and so on, often speak louder and more forcefully than words.

Listening is also *active* in that it hears what is not spoken but implied. 'Can't you do something more for this pain?' may in reality be saying 'You are not taking my pain seriously and I am angry with you for this'. The implication is the anger. Written on paper it may sound flat, but combined with the patient's tone of voice and the look in his or her eyes, it is a different matter.

What is this person trying to communicate? What is he saying about his feelings? What is he saying with his behaviour? Why is he saying it now and what does it mean?

To *hear* another person is perhaps the biggest gift we can ever give. When you hear someone, you accept him or her unconditionally, without any judgement. When you hear individuals, you give them the means to hear themselves. Carkhuff described counselling to be for growth; psychotherapy talks about becoming. When you listen in such a way that your clients can hear themselves, then they are able to become themselves, and to grow.

Listening is active in that it listens *for* something. It listens for the person, for all that she or he expresses. It listens in particular for the feelings expressed or hidden. It listens for the meaning which all this may have for the person. It listens finally for a goal to emerge, and for ways in which the person can or could change.

You don't keep this to yourself. The essence of empathy is that you hear the other and communicate this back so that you both know that understanding has taken place.

Patient: And if anything happens to him, well, Lord knows what will happen to me. Shoved in a home for geriatrics I suppose. But I mustn't look on that side of things.

Nurse: But you do look on that side. I heard you say things about being useless several times.

Patient: Well, this is it. I do feel useless, and I have never been useless in my life, but, the only thing is, if I can't be useful because I am immobile, then perhaps I can be useful in other ways. There is a nurse over there who has got marital problems, and she was showering me the other day and I got talking to her, and she said I helped. And I thought, well, if I can help people that way it won't be so bad, will it? I shan't be completely useless.

When you listen to the other you are less inclined to listen to yourself. You are then not making statements like 'You should do what I did . . .'. In that instance you are not hearing the needs of the other, but your own, relating what you hear to yourself. When you are listening to another person you filter what is said through you.

You let the words drip *through* you like water; you don't divert the water into your channel.

Patient: Sister, I know I shouldn't be saying this, but I just can't get on with Nurse N. Can't you give me another one to look after me?

Nurse: You don't get on with N.?

Patient: She is rude to me.

Nurse: Can you be more specific?

Patient: She always calls me 'little Doris'. I told her I am not 'little'.

Nurse: She diminishes you.

Patient: Yes, she makes me feel a child. She treats me as if I were a nitwit.

Nurse: You are saying that with pain in your voice.

Patient: (bursts into tears) I've been trying so hard all my life to do the right thing. Somehow, she has managed to get where it hurts most.

Nurse: What does doing the right thing mean for you?

Patient: Do you really want to listen to a long story?

Nurse: Sounds like you need to tell it – go on please.

This edited and shortened form of a conversation (which did not finish where the extract ends) shows several of the points made in this chapter: the full acceptance of the client without judging her or diverting from her subject. The nurse gave her the space and time she needed. The many 'um's and 'ah's and pauses used would make this point more clearly. She gave her permission to talk. She encouraged her; she helped her to get to her own strong point: 'doing the right thing'. With that she was into the area of meaning for and in her life. And so the process repeats itself: attention calls forth permission to talk, encouragement and empowerment.

Listening (like the wise old owl) is hearing a great deal, and often not saying much. (A posture can sometimes say just as much.) Perhaps a pragmatic way of translating the little rhyme could be:

Nature gave man two ears but only one tongue, which is a gentle hint, that he should listen more than he talks. (Davis, 1972)

8 Counselling skills: exploring

Exploring
'The task of counselling is to give the client an opportunity to explore, discover and clarify ways of living more satisfyingly and resourcefully' (British Association for Counselling, 1984). Exploration is the first step on this road, and it is often a lengthy and sometimes painful road. With the exploration goes discovery. Frankl (1962) believes that meaning is only ever *discovered*, not created, by a person. In order to discover that meaning, a considerable amount of exploring has to be done.

Exploring the inner world of a person is not unlike exploring a completely uncharted land. You have no maps, no roads, no signposts. You probably only have a compass. That compass is the person's inner strength or potential which steadily points in the direction of fulfilment. You have a model, or theoretical framework, which could be analogous to the daily routine and survival tactics of an explorer.

Among these tactics are certain skills, which those who do a lot of exploring perhaps don't think about much any more, but people new to the discipline need to learn. Some of these skills are outlined here. There are many more available, and necessary at times, depending on the skills, or lack of them, of the helper or the client, and depending on the problem.

So far, I have referred mainly to the skills of the helper. The fact is that the client also needs skills. He or she may have these already but they may need sharpening. Or they may indeed be lacking. They are, in particular, the skills of self-help but also include basic social skills, mainly skills of relating and assertiveness.

Allowing

One of the most 'obvious' skills in helping is giving permission. That is what it is about: 'I give you permission to talk'. But it is not necessarily so obvious. Helpers often take it for granted that they give permission; clients often dare not take the permission, so it has to be spelled out. Giving the permission to talk, and allowing someone to then tell his or her story is basic to helping.

Fabun (1968) believes that no experience ever begins. There was always something that went before. The only thing that begins is the person's awareness of something going on. In a sense, therefore, every story always begins with 'and'. This can be infuriating for those people who like things neatly wrapped up but it can be liberating for those who know that they can never really reach an end, only a new beginning.

This little word 'and' is also the word of relationships: 'You and me'; 'I and Thou'. It is the word which most of us need to learn to say more sincerely.

Allowing individuals to tell their story is an opening of yourself to each person which is based on affirming both yourself and the other. On this affirmation the desire to change can be built.

This story-telling is the first stage of any problem definition (Egan); the **D**escribe (Nelson-Jones) part of helping. Very often the client does not know what the problem actually is, or is not sufficiently in touch with it. So that the problem can be described and defined, the story may have to be described in considerable detail; or it may have to be taken back further and further – more and more 'ands' have to be added. This may mean going down memory lanes, up garden paths, through long, dark corridors, opening doors here and there, looking around corners and turning over every stone. No wonder our language is full of such images!

In that telling, things are not only clarified but also healed. Most bereaved persons have to tell the story of the death or illness many times over. Each telling of the story allows some details to be changed, emerge, or be dropped, and in that change it becomes more part of the person. 'The outer journey is the plot; the inner journey is the meaning' (Navone, 1977).

Some people have no particular sense of journey. They see life as a succession of events which happen to them. In being allowed to tell the story of these events, shapes may begin to emerge, patterns can begin to be recognized, and links can be made between happenings which never seemed to be related. In this way some meaning which lay hidden for years may begin to emerge. These meanings are often the strong points in a person's life which help him to keep going, sometimes against all odds. They are what makes a person 'tick'.

The skills which the helper needs are those of giving permission to talk, encouraging the continuation of the story-telling, being unafraid of what she might hear, and listening for that which matters and has meaning in the person's life.

The client too has to be unafraid: unafraid of actually telling the story. Some people feel that their story is so awful that they dare not repeat it. If they want to be helped then they have to say what they need help with.

Peter was an 18-year-old with suspected cancer of the testes. He asked his nurse to tell him what the prognosis was for this kind of cancer.

Nurse: I could give you facts and figures. Is that what you want?
Peter: Not only.
Nurse: How else can I help you?
Peter: Well, I wondered . . . You see, I am . . . Oh, I can't really tell you . . . .
Nurse: It's all right, tell me what you can. I'll do the same.

The nurse was not quite sure why Peter had asked that particular question as she knew Peter was well informed about tests and treatments, so her question is directed to the *person*, not just the problem. To allow him to say a bit more, she was therefore deliberately open at the beginning. By saying later that she, too, will tell Peter as much as she can, she made a kind of 'pact' with Peter to collaborate, and that may have given Peter the security to be as open as possible.

If the nurse had simply concentrated on the 'problem' presented, i.e. the prognosis, she might have said something like

Nurse: That depends on many things and it's too early to be sure at this moment.

Peter would probably never have said anything more.

Allowing means allowing 'things' to happen. In this case the nurse got quite a story.

Seeking information   Much of counselling, particularly in the early stages, depends on information. As a helper you need a fair amount of information to help effectively. The client is helped by telling his story, hearing himself recount what happened or how things are.

When seeking information, the most obvious tool to use is questioning. But questions are not always appropriate, as they can let the client do less work and rely only on questions. Much information can be sought without asking questions. You can use statements like, 'You said that it hurts you to say that – I am not sure if I quite understood that', or 'You feel trapped in your situation at work. Maybe you could tell me more about being trapped', or 'I see that taking that action is risky. I can't quite relate this to what you said earlier about it being exciting'.

You may have to ask for further information when a client's story is unclear. What seems clear to the client may not be so clear to anybody else. The types of questions you ask, and how you ask them, will be crucial for the information you get.

A look at questions in general is therefore called for.

According to Tomlinson (1983) the functions of questions are:

1. Gathering information.
2. Encouraging conversation.
3. Identifying problems and difficulties.
4. Focusing attention on specific issues or topics.
5. Expressing interest in others.
6. Discovering attitudes and opinions of others.

The skill of questioning is in the way questions and behaviour, tone and attitude, blend. The following are types of questions as categorized by Hargie et al (1981):

1. Recall
2. Process
3. Closed
4. Open
5. Affective
6. Leading
7. Probing
8. Rhetorical
9. Multiple.

Recall questions These questions involve only remembering information. They are commonly used at the beginning of interviews:

What is your name?
When did you first go to the doctor?

Process questions These involve more complex mental processes. Process questions ask for opinions, judgements, analysis and interpretation of situations, and are used to encourage people to think more deeply about a subject:

Why do you think it is important to learn about questions?
What are the characteristics of a good nurse?

Closed questions Closed questions place restrictions on the respondent. There is usually only one correct answer. They give the questioner control over the situation and they provide focus. Such questions are generally:

1. *Selective* (either/or):
   Do you prefer tea or coffee?
2. *Yes/no*:
   Did you have a good night?
3. *Identification of the past, present or future*:
   When are you taking your holiday?

Open questions Open questions leave the respondent free to answer as he wishes. They are broad in nature, but are more time-consuming, and answers may contain irrelevant but valuable and unexpected information. They encourage the respondent to talk, leaving the questioner free to observe, listen and learn.

Tell me about your spare-time activities.
What's it like being so far from home?

Affective questions These allow people to discuss emotions, feelings and attitudes, and within this can be recall, process, closed or open questions.

How do you feel about this news?
In what ways have your feelings changed since then?

Leading questions They lead the respondent towards an expected reply by the way they are worded. The leads can be simple or subtle, they can convey friendliness, or can imply things.

Isn't it a lovely day?
Surely you don't believe this sort of thing?

Probing questions These questions are designed to encourage the respondent to enlarge or expand on the initial responses. They are often of the follow-up type.

Can you explain what you mean?
And then what happened?

Rhetorical questions Rhetorical questions do not always expect an answer, either because the speaker intends to answer, or because the question is equivalent to a statement.

Who would not wish their children well?

Multiple questions These are where two or more questions are phrased in one; they are very confusing, especially to the elderly. It also means that often only the last question is answered, and the others are forgotten or overlooked.

Have you lived here long? Do you like it? I mean, what are the neighbours like?
Good morning Mr Smith. Would you like a cup of tea and a wash? (Tomlinson, 1983; Tschudin, 1989c)

All these types of questions will be used at one time or another in helping situations. You are not only seeking facts, but you are seeking to understand the world of your client. From this point of view, perhaps the most useful types of questions are the open questions and the affective questions. In order to help, you need to direct the client to disclose herself, and that means mainly her feelings. Once you have concentrated on the feelings, you need to help the search for meaning.

What do you feel about it?
What are you feeling now?
What is the meaning of it?

Patient: It had been such a blow to me then.
Nurse: What do you think that blow means to you now?
Patient: (silence) It had never occurred to me to look at it in terms of meaning. I wish someone would have asked me that question twenty years ago, it would have clarified a lot!

Reflecting

Reflecting is perhaps the most widely known and useful skill of helping.

Reflecting means throwing something back and causing it to rebound. In using reflecting as a skill, you are giving back to the client the very words he has just used. This is the basic use of this skill.

There is also a more advanced use of reflection, in that

you give back that which was *not* there but was implied.

Patient: I can't use the time the way I would like to. That's the worst part.

Nurse: It seems as if wasting time is something that is an important issue for you.

Patient: I could do a lot of reading, but I can't read. And I could prepare work, but it just packs in on me. I can't think, and people say to me, it's about time you laid back and thought a while.

Nurse: It sounds as if you are finding your own company quite difficult.

For this patient 'wasting time' was the problem which he could talk about, but underneath lay the difficulty of not accepting his illness. In this interaction both types of reflection are illustrated.

When you stay with the patient at the level of the words he uses, you stay with him where the problem lies. This means repeating the important word, or concept, and giving it back to him so that *he* can *hear* what he has just said.

Patient: But I was so desperate to find an answer, and if possible an easy one. I thought, ah well, it's just a little lump in the elbow and they can just remove it and all will be well.

Nurse: You were desperate though.

A psychiatric patient repeatedly said that she *must* change her attitude. She constantly made plans for changing her environment, believing that everything would then be all right. This usually worked for a few days, then her environment was again not conducive to changing her attitudes. She sought help from all who came into contact with her but usually rejected the help offered.

Patient: I really need to get through this. I am on the brink of losing everything and it's just . . . .

Nurse: Stop a minute. You just said something important there. You said 'I need to get through this'.

Patient: (slowly) Yes, I must get through this.

Nurse: You said, 'I *need* to get through'.

Patient: Did I?

Nurse: You said 'need'.

Patient: Yes, sure, I must get through it, how else will it work?

Nurse: You *need* to.

Patient: I need to.

Nurse: There is a great deal of difference between needing to and must.

Patient: What is it?

This patient was gradually helped to see that by acknowledging her *need* she was willing to be helped, whereas her own *must* was a kind of pulling herself up by her own boot-straps, which was not possible for her.

This interaction shows that sometimes reflecting just the one word which matters will bring a person to the necessary insight.

The following is an extract from a discussion with a patient in a rehabilitation unit where he had gone after a spell in another hospital.

Patient: In the other hospital there was a group of us at one stage and we got on incredibly well. But that's different here.

Nurse: Are you saying that you are lonely?

Patient: Oh no, not lonely. But I do miss talking over the problems from school every day with my wife (they were both teachers). Discussing and working things out together.

Nurse: You are missing something – something you identify with.

Patient: Talking and discussing has always been something I identified with.

In this interaction the reflecting done by the helper is of the second kind: reflecting what may only be implied. This is the type of empathy which is so valuable in helping a person to come to understand himself, and what to do with this understanding. In this way the problems may begin to be acknowledged and described, and goals may emerge.

If this is to happen, then the skill of reflecting is not used only by the helper. The client too, has to do a good deal of reflecting: of his situation, his problem, his perception, his attitudes, beliefs and values. But this reflection is perhaps more of the type of thought and 'going back over' than throwing back. It is a reconsideration, rather than a rebounding.

Clarifying

The goal of helping is to enable the client to live more effectively. Many of the helping situations which we meet start out with the client being very unclear: 'I don't know what's the matter with me, but I'm not feeling very well today'. The initial goal of helping is to clarify what is going on. Unless the client is clear what the problem is, decisions as to what to do about it cannot be made.

The first response to an unclear statement is therefore often one of clarification.

In what way are you not feeling well?
Can you tell me what it is you *are* feeling?

After some initial unfolding of the problem, the more important issues can then be elucidated. Any problem situation is made up of experiences, behaviours and feelings, and active listening will help to clarify these. Helping becomes useful only when there are specific things to concentrate on.

Clarifying is making clear: to yourself as helper; to the client what he is meaning; and as a first step towards a goal.

One of the ways in which counselling is diminished is by making assumptions.

Patient: I have always had difficulties with my mother.
Nurse: (This is obviously a regression problem)

Patient: I am never sure how to spell that word.
Nurse: (She must be dyslexic)

Moorey and Greer (1989) show an interesting example of how easily assumptions can get everything wrong:

After a mastectomy a young woman lost interest in sex. She felt depressed and lethargic. Her negative thoughts centred on her disturbed body image: 'I am so completely unattractive that he can't possibly want me any more'.
When her husband made a sexual approach she rebuffed him, thinking: 'He's only being sympathetic, he can't really want me'.
Unaware of her automatic thoughts her husband became prey to thoughts of his own: 'Her sexual feelings have disappeared. She's frigid'. He gave up making sexual advances. (see p. 107)

Before you make a decision in your own mind that your client is this or that sort of person, or that you know exactly what his problem is, check it out.

Patient: I have always had difficulties with my mother.
Nurse: Can you tell me of some of the difficulties you have with your mother?

This does not only help you to know more precisely

what the problem is; it will also help the client to spell out, perhaps for the first time, what had until then only been an amorphous mass which could not be controlled. By looking at it in more detail, with more clarity, it may become less overwhelming and more manageable.

Some examples of how to clarify are:

Patient: I'm not very well today.
Nurse: In what way are you not well?

Patient: I don't know what's going on with me.
Nurse: Can you be more specific?

Patient: I am not in control of myself.
Nurse: What does it mean for you to be in control of yourself?

Patient: It will be alright in the end.
Nurse: What in particular will be alright?

Patient: Things keep going wrong.
Nurse: What sort of things keep going wrong?

Summarizing

Egan (1982) sees summarizing primarily as a 'bridging-skill' between the various stages. This is certainly true, but it can also bridge other aspects of the helping process.

The technique of making a summary in helping can focus scattered thoughts and feelings. It can also close the conversation on a particular theme, or it can prompt the client to explore a particular theme more thoroughly (Brammer, 1973). A summary should present the relevant facts.

Nurse: From what you have said, I can detect three points: you had had all the tests and they were all negative. Nevertheless, you have a pain which persists. You think it's linked with something from the past but you are afraid to look into the past. Is this correct?

A summary can be a mixture of what was said and implied. Summarizing is a 'directing' skill. When the client is directionless, as is quite frequent early on, this skill helps to gather the situation together. Also, in the early stages there is necessarily a lot of information passed between the two people, and some of it may be confused, or with gaps in it which are clear to the client, but not the helper. Making a summary can then help you from getting lost in either too few or too many details.

The skill of summarizing has also a quality of 'where do we go from here?' about it. It is therefore a very good tactic to use, either when the client or the session is 'stuck' or getting nowhere. To make a summary of what has gone on so far may help to give the larger picture by pulling the various topics together. Once a larger but more precise picture is available, this can act like a springboard for further work.

Summarizing, according to Brammer (1973), is mainly useful in giving the client a sense of movement. It is therefore also particularly useful at the end of a session. So often when an insight is gained or something is seen in a new light, the effect of this is lost because it is not noticed. Therefore, at the end of a conversation you can make a short summary of the main topics covered or insights gained. When they are thus gathered in a few words or sentences, they can be held more easily, thought about, and used in the next days or weeks. What is thus captured is less easily lost again, and helps you to see where you have come from. However, summarizing is no substitute for further exploration of an anxiety-provoking topic. The object of summarizing is not to package up something unsightly or painful but to point things out in all their various aspects or guises.

Dealing with feelings

Quite simply, we are what we feel. Someone who is not feeling happy *is* not happy. And it is not just the mood which is not happy; the whole body is not happy. If we want to help people in a holistic way, we have to take all aspects of this seriously.

Dealing with a person's feelings is not easy. Many people mix up feelings and thinking. You ask them 'How do you feel about this?' and they answer 'I think . . .'.

Feelings are as varied as life itself. There are the generally recognizable feelings of fear, anger, sadness, despair, joy, embarrassment, love, frustration, and so on. But there are many other feelings which have no particular name, and of which everybody is differently aware. There are levels or degrees of feelings. Being pleased is weaker than being excited, though it is still a feeling of happiness (Tschudin, 1989b).

Feelings and emotional states can lead people to maintain attitudes and behave in ways which restrict their lives and diminish their potential. They affect their lives and cloud their judgements.

'When troubled emotions appear to be taking over, there is a tendency to "send for the expert"' (Scrutton, 1989). We ask for the pain to be taken away. But, unlike pain, feelings cannot be removed with pills. It is only when the individual owns the feelings and takes responsibility for them that they can be dealt with. It is only when we can be in charge of our feelings, rather than they being in charge of us, that we can begin to live satisfyingly and resourcefully. Only then can we begin to fulfil our potential.

Thus, dealing with a person's feelings is a fundamental aspect of helping. When you do that, you are dealing with the person, not the problem.

The often-recurring questions must therefore be:
What are you feeling about that?
How do you feel now?
What does that bring up in the way of feelings?
Have you always felt like that?
Where in your body do you feel this (fear, anger)?
Do you have other feelings besides this one?
When do you feel like this particularly?

Look at the following discussion with a patient and look out particularly for the feelings mentioned and how they were dealt with.

Patient: Do you think that death is as taboo a subject now as sex in Victorian times?

Nurse: Probably, yes.

Patient: I have to make a confession: I have never seen a dead body, not even my father when he died. I rationalize it; I was afraid.

Nurse: How do you feel about death now?

Patient: I'm afraid of pain. If I have to die . . ..

Nurse: You are afraid of pain?

Patient: More than death, actually. The thought of pain – I'd do anything to be rid of it.

Nurse: What sort of pain are you afraid of?

Patient: Nagging pain.

Nurse: Nagging pain?

Patient: Nag, nag, nag, all day, without relief.

Nurse: Like the boss you just told me about.

Patient: Funny – yes, I hadn't made the connection.

When you can stop and stay with the feelings, then all sorts of doors will open. The vista opening up may not always be of glorious sunshine; it can often be a dense fog, or dark night. But the reward for facing whatever is presented in this way may be a glorious dawn, one day.

The other important thing at this point is that you, as the helper, go with your client into the 'weather' outside. This is what helping is about. You are the companion on the road and that is a more real and fulfilling way to be human than to swallow a pill to kill pain. When clients know that you are there, they may begin to take responsibility for their feelings and thus trust themselves, and you, to change some of the inhibiting attitudes and behaviours.

Some people are very little in touch with their feelings; with relationships particularly, they will deny that they have any feelings:

One man, who was in hospital for a short spell during a long-term illness, learnt that his wife had left him for his next-door neighbour. When asked how he felt, he repeatedly replied 'I don't feel anything. She walked out'.

He *may* not have been feeling anything because he was shocked (see p. 26) and numbed but, deeper than that, he denied having any responsibility in his wife's decision to leave.

When someone is in a state of shock it is not possible to do any 'real' counselling. This is not what the person usually needs anyway. What is needed is nurture, and that consists of *giving* good things, like tempting and easily-digested food for a convalescent person, encouragement, rebuilding the self-image, and fostering trust. When the person is more secure, the more solid 'food' can be given again: the reflecting and challenging which are necessary for growth, self-responsibility and self-help.

Sometimes people find it simply impossible to talk about their feelings. Fraser (1990) has shown that by encouraging her pregnant clients to write down their feelings as letters or stories she was able to help them significantly by reading the lines, and between them, to discover what mattered most. This is a possibility which could also be used in many other settings.

Self-sharing   Self-sharing is not the same type of skill as that just outlined, but it is mentioned here because it is often very helpful at this exploratory stage. Clients can see any helpers, including nurses, as experts, and thus 'above' them. Additionally, many people feel very isolated with their feelings and think that they alone in the whole, wide world suffer the particular problem and that nobody can understand them. When you can gently undo these assumptions by telling the client something about yourself, then you have achieved a great deal.

Self-sharing is a way of 'being with' your client:

> Yes, I was once in a similar situation to you, and I can remember feeling almost the same as you are saying now: a feeling of loneliness and being abandoned. Perhaps such feelings are an area we could work on now.

One difficulty with self-sharing is that it can become 'I know exactly how you feel!'. With the best empathy in the world you will never know *exactly* how someone else feels. A mother of a stillborn baby or a bereaved person might be particularly hurt by such a statement.

When you use this skill, try to be tentative but realistic, careful but not apologetic. Notice what difference it makes to a client if you offer something of yourself. The aim is to allow the client to go on talking more about a personal problem. Self-sharing is only useful if it encourages this.

Patient: I always say the wrong thing at the wrong time.
Nurse: I have so often felt like that too! I always feel such a fool then, and I guess that is how you are feeling too.

Self-sharing can be tremendously liberating. Suddenly you feel equals, two human beings with each other, but the aim of self-sharing is not that *you* feel better, but that your client can move forward and perhaps feel less isolated. You are now truly his *companion*, that is, 'the one who shares bread with him'. The image is a strong one. And as usual, these images contain much truth. You *share* your bread; you don't give it all. In so doing he too may learn to share, and that is essentially what living is all about.

These skills of exploring are not only used at the beginning of a helping relationship, they are used throughout.

There may be a hint in these chapters about skills that helping is a long-term relationship. It can be that. It is also possible for helping to last only a few minutes. The skills and the process are the same, as indeed I hope some of the interactions show.

9 *Empathy*

Defining empathy

The word empathy is used a great deal these days; like the word counselling, it is often used and understood wrongly. To help give it its rightful place, a short chapter on this basic 'ingredient' for helping is therefore indicated.

Rogers (1957) was the first to use the term empathy as part of therapy. Later (1959) he used the following definition: empathy is 'the ability to perceive the internal frame of reference of another with accuracy, and with the emotional components and meaning which pertain thereto, as if one were the other person, but without ever losing the "as if" condition'.

A shorter, and more cogent definition is that used by Kalisch (1971): 'Empathy is the ability to perceive accurately the feelings of another person and to communicate this understanding to him'. This definition points to the two-way nature of empathy: understanding the other person, and reflecting that understanding to him. It is not enough for the helper to understand a client, the client also needs to be helped by this understanding.

Mayeroff (1972) describes this understanding in a philosophical way, and from the point of view of caring:

To care for another person I must be able to understand him and his world as if I were inside it. I must be able to see, as it were, with his eyes what his world is like to him and how he sees himself. Instead of merely looking at him in a detached way from outside, as if he were a specimen, I must be able to be *with* him in his world, 'going' into into his world in order to sense from 'inside' what life is like for him, what he is striving to be, and what he requires to grow.

Empathy or sympathy?

The following allegory may highlight the difference between empathy and sympathy.

A person has fallen into a ditch, and is unable to get out of it. A *sympathetic* person comes along, sees the victim, goes to him and lies in the ditch with him, and both talk of this terrible misadventure and of other similar ones they had both experienced in the past. An *unsympathetic* person comes along the road, sees the person lying there and shouts to him 'Don't just lie there, pull yourself together, do something!' But the victim has broken bones, and he cannot move, and the helper neither sees nor hears what the victim is saying because he is standing too far away. An *empathic* person who comes that way climbs down to the victim and gives what first aid is necessary. Then he listens to what the victim has to say, how the accident happened, what led up to it, and what he now feels and experiences. This helper is completely present, but figuratively he has one foot on the bank, the firm ground. This eventually enables him to help the victim get out of the ditch on to his own legs, and to the way he wants to go, the way which is right for him.

To begin with, many helping situations need some practical help: information, the right form to fill in or a telephone call. Equally, to begin with, a person may 'just' need to talk and be heard. Anyone shocked and numbed needs nurturing, not counselling. 'Tea and sympathy' is not such a bad thing, as long as you keep one foot on the firm ground and change to empathy when the moment is right.

Daniel (1984) distinguishes empathy from sympathy by saying that the prefix 'em' corresponds to 'en' or 'in', as in insight or intuition, whereas in sympathy the prefix 'sym' corresponds to 'syn' or 'like'. Empathy, she says, 'is an intuitive leap of mind and feeling which encompasses all the aspects and the condition of the sufferer'. Empathy is deeper than sympathy, because it goes 'in' and uses imagination. Sympathy, being 'like', cannot make that leap of 'sensitive receptivity to the suffering of another' because it is too much tied to the self. Sympathy compares with another; insight is achieved only with empathy.

Being empathic

What then is empathy? How is it expressed, recognized, communicated?

Both Carkhuff (1969) and Egan (1982) speak of two levels of empathy. In first-level empathy the helper responds to the words spoken and reflects them: she communicates an initial, basic understanding, as in this dialogue between patient and nurse.

Patient: I feel really terrible today, worse than yesterday.
Nurse: You feel worse today?

The *words* are repeated, or reflected. This is the basic act of empathy: the helper shows that the client is heard. She acknowledges that hearing by going no further than the client, and staying at the same level as the client. Responding to the words spoken is the initial essential step in helping.

Patient: I feel really terrible today, worse than yesterday.
Nurse: Don't worry, these things take time.

This nurse has heard the words, and is responding to the implication, but inappropriately, not empathically. After such an interaction there is nothing more for a client to say. The nurse has indicated that she doesn't want to hear anything further. This is clearly an unempathic remark.

The first simple response to the words shows that the helper wants to hear more. She is ready to listen. She starts, in the image of the story, to climb down to the victim; she makes the first move towards him. Responding to the words spoken is, in Egan's (1982) terms, 'primary-level accurate empathy'. The information which the client gives is received by the helper who, in responding with the same words as those used by the client, shows that she has heard. At the same time this is also a check that she has heard correctly. Essentially the skill of reflecting (see Chapter 8) is used here.

This primary level may be used initially, in the first few exchanges of a conversation. When enough information has been given and received, the helper should then move onto the second stage, 'advanced accurate empathy'. There is less reflection of words, but more of feelings, of implied behaviours, and of underlying trends. At this level, intuition and 'hunches' play a role, and there is some interpretation going on. This second, deeper level of empathy picks out the unspoken feeling or reason behind what is said.

Patient: I feel terrible today, worse than yesterday.
Nurse: You sound dejected at feeling worse today.

Both levels of empathy are necessary. In most interactions there is a certain amount of initial information giving and receiving before the conversation can go deeper. The helper who listens well will have taken any such cues from the client, and not have offered them unsolicited.

Recognizing two levels of empathy is useful for training and learning purposes. Once a person uses them they will become quite spontaneous. It is important to realize that in any interaction both levels of empathy are generally used side by side. To begin with, the primary level is used most, going on to the second level gradually. If only the primary level is used, a client may still reach her goal, but more slowly and laboriously, or the conversation may grind to a halt, because no *helping* is actually done, even though reflection may take place.

Even when using advanced empathy it is helpful and useful to come back to simple reflection and to first-level empathy. The two levels need to be used side by side. A primary-level response is often necessary to check something out: 'Is that the right feeling?' or 'Was that what you said?' or 'Am I right in thinking . . .?'.

Patient: I can't use the time the way I would like to. That's the worst part.

Nurse: Is that what is bothering you?

Patient: Yes, the fact that I can't use the time profitably . . . I suppose basically I am not a man of action.

Nurse: You are not a man of action?

Patient: No. That surprises you?

Nurse: It does surprise me.

Patient: I am . . . what am I?

Empathy is *the* basis for helping. It takes the first step and then keeps going further and further towards the client. But it is not only something we *do*; it is also something we *are*.

Scales for measuring empathy exist (Truax, 1961; Carkhuff, 1969; Hogan, 1969). What they measure is generally the empathic communication, i.e. the accuracy of the response given by the helper. It is much more difficult to measure the benefits or results of empathy. Forsyth (1979) found that when she measured patients' perception of empathy, the results were distorted because they rated all nurses as empathic, probably for fear of giving bad marks to students. She also noted that 'nurses can make empathic remarks without experiencing empathy. Perhaps that is the meaning of the finding that clients' perceptions of psychiatric nurses' empathy is high, while actually the nurses' empathic abilities are lower than expected'. Empathy is more than words: it is 'being' and 'being with'.

It is this latter, this 'being with', which Rogers emphasized more and more as the only condition for helping. He rarely spoke of empathy as 'the right thing to say'; he described empathy as 'a very special way of being' (Rogers, 1975). In his last book *A Way of Being* (1980) he wrote his 'current definition' which contains some of the following statements:

An empathic way of being with another person . . . means entering the private perceptual world of the other and becoming thoroughly at home in it. It involves being sensitive . . . without making judgements . . . communicating your sensings of the person's world as you look with fresh and unfrightened eyes at elements of which he or she is fearful . . . In some sense it means that you lay aside your self . . . being empathic is a complex, demanding, and strong – yet also a subtle and gentle – way of being.

Empathy is the basis of helping, and any skills are built on this basis. Empathy is a skill, but it is also more than a skill. The following quotation shows empathy in action.

A colleague has recently described to me an occasion when a West Indian woman in a London flat was told of her husband's death in a street accident. The shock of the grief stunned her like a blow, she sank into a corner of the sofa and sat there rigid and unhearing. For a long time her terrible tranced look continued to embarrass the family, friends and officials who came and went. Then the schoolteacher of one of her children, an Englishwoman, called, and seeing how things were, went and sat beside her. Without a word she threw an arm around the tight shoulders, clasping them with her full strength. The white cheek was thrust hard against the brown. Then as the unrelenting pain seeped through to her, the newcomer's tears began to flow, falling on their two hands linked in the woman's lap. For a long time that is all that was happening. And then at last the West Indian woman started to sob. Still not a word was spoken and after a little while the visitor got up and went, leaving her contribution to help the family meet its immediate needs (Taylor, 1972)

10 Counselling skills: goal setting

What is your goal?

Counselling is goal oriented, and all the help given to a person is therefore given with the aim of reaching a goal. It can be compared with a tree: its essence is the fruit (the goal) and the budding and flowering beforehand, the listening and exploring. All are necessary, but one without the other is wasteful.

When you are listening to a person's story (when the tree is budding) you begin to get an idea of who and what this person is. When you explore together what all this may mean (when the tree is flowering) you get a wide picture of what has been, what is now present, and what might emerge. When you search for and discuss a goal or goals then your work for the tree is bearing fruit.

Egan (1986) says that 'counselling is a process of helping clients become more *intentional*'. Individual clients are in an uncomfortable situation now, but with your help they are moving to a more comfortable way of being. They have for one reason or another lost their intention in life and ask you to help them regain it or find a different or more appropriate intention. This intention, according to Egan, includes 'self-responsibility, a refusal to buckle, a sense of direction, versatility and the ability to transcend self-interest'.

A sense of direction and versatility are the main aspects of the skills of goal setting.

New perspectives

In order to find the direction or goal in which to move, a person needs to have various possibilities. To be effective as a human being, he has to make choices, and these are only possible when there are alternatives. The process of goal setting is thus a process of choosing from alternatives, or seeing the best way forward from among a variety.

In the story of the person in the ditch (Chapter 9), the empathic helper keeps one foot on the firm ground. Not both, just one. It is the one foot with the client which conveys that you are there too, and the one foot outside which gives you a certain distance, allowing you to step in and step out to help the person. You do not present the client with the goal, but you may point to certain possibilities which may give your client a choice. For that one purpose you are like a shop assistant, displaying various products for the client to look at, perhaps try out, and then choose to buy.

The skills of helping may be described in the shape of a diamond. At the bottom point is the client: narrow, stuck, and unable to move. As he tells his or her story, the shape becomes wider upwards and more open to different influences. At its widest point are all the different options, which then have to be narrowed again into the point at the top: the goal, or aim. Helping to be in touch with an increasing number of perspectives is the basis for goal setting. This can be achieved by a variety of means.

Imagination

The helping skills outlined so far have concentrated on what is happening now and on what has gone before to bring a person to the present state. Essentially, helping is for the future: what life might be like from now on. That has to do with imagination. We cannot *know* the future; we can only imagine it. In the process of goal setting, this is the client's best tool for moving towards the top of the figurative diamond.

Many people feel that imagination is kids' stuff and that to be adult is to be rational. Rogers (1978) quotes research done on senior level managers which showed that the most effective and productive managers of enterprises were able to 'engage in personal fantasy, daydreams, fictional speculations . . . think and associate to ideas in unusual ways, have unconventional thought processes . . . (are) skilled in social techniques of imaginative play, pretending, and humour'.

Clients are stuck, or in a morass, precisely because they cannot imagine how to get out of it. If they did, they wouldn't need help.

When the moment in helping for the situation to be

shaped and anchored has been reached, then the important question 'What would your world look like if it were a little better?' may be crucial. The operative word is 'little'. In the nature of things we tend to go from the sublime to the ridiculous, and from being stuck we want things to be perfect. That is not actually helpful because it becomes quickly evident that too much all at once is impossible, and even self-defeating. By asking for a little imagination you are helping the client to move from the present scenario (Egan) to the preferred scenario, one step at a time.

The mother of 24-year-old Christopher with Down's syndrome was at the end of her tether when the district nurse called by chance. She was looking after him single handed. He had another attack of bronchitis and she was afraid this would turn into pneumonia.

Mother: It's times like this that get me down. I am totally tied up with him, and then I realize that I have no life of my own.

Nurse: You are feeling resentful of life?

Mother: You could say that.

Nurse: It's difficult never to do your own thing.

Mother: I've turned all the possibilities over and over in my mind and there is no solution that I would be happy with other than caring for him myself.

Nurse: The question may not be a solution, but something to aim for.

Mother: How do you mean?

Nurse: I mean, how would your life be if it were just a little better? Not perfect, just a little better?

Mother: I would see more of my friends, . . . get that degree . . .

Sometimes a question like this can be mistaken. The answer in this case might have been something like:

Mother: I would be free and Christopher would not be handicapped.

The important thing is to put the question in such a way that it is not heard as asking for 'the world', but asking for the possible.

Notice also how the nurse addressed the mother and her life, not the 'problem'. That gave her the possibility to be imaginative rather than seeking a solution.

This points to the other use of imagination: it comes from the person himself. It is not something imposed. This helps to make a goal more realistic and self-chosen.

The responsibility for the goal is more directly with the client.

Imagination can be used in a great variety of situations.

Helper: What would you have liked to have said to him?
Client: I am not your servant.

Helper: What could you change that you haven't changed so far?
Client: I could go to work there on Tuesdays rather than Wednesdays.

Helper: What decisions could you take now rather than wait?
Client: I could make contact with her now, then I would know where I stand in relation to her to begin with.

It cannot be stressed enough that the aim of helping is that the client is able to manage his or her life more resourcefully and satisfyingly. This means that there is a goal, a direction or purpose evident. For this to become evident, there needs to be some exploration and clarification. But there may not necessarily be a great deal of self-analysis and insight into the problems of living. Once a person can manage a direction, then self-analysis will happen 'by the way', so to speak. The use of the imagination for finding the goal or direction is therefore not only vital but can actually also be refreshingly new, and fun.

Intuition

In contrast to the client's use of imagination, you the helper can put new perspectives on the table by your use of intuition, hunches and 'sixth sense'.

As helper, you are deeply involved with the helped person. In such a relationship you too have your ideas, insights and memories which relate to what is going on now. But whereas the client is stuck, you are not. You see possibilities for moving forward. You make connections where the client hadn't made them. You see patterns which the client is blind to. These, too, can help the client to see a wider picture. The skill lies in the way you present these pictures from your view so that they broaden the view of the other, rather than blot it out.

A hunch, an insight, an intuition is 'an involuntary event, which depends upon different external or internal circumstances, instead of an act of judgement'. (Jung 1964)

Ferrucci (1982) puts this in a practical way:

Intuition perceives *wholes*, while our everyday analytical mind is used to dealing with *parts* and therefore finds the synthesizing grasp of the intuition unfamiliar. But after an intuition does appear, it may even seem to us to have revealed something obvious; we ask, 'why haven't I seen this before?'

When you use your intuition for helping it becomes a kind of challenge. The client is jolted out of a narrow view of the self and the surrounding world around into a wider view. Bridges suddenly appear where there were none, and what is more, the person is also enabled to cross them.

Intuition is not only a helper skill; the client can use it too. Helping goes on beyond the time spent with a person. When each has been opened to awareness, all sorts of places, words, pictures and dreams may give insights, and intuitively reveal the self to the self.

As a helper you may or may not be at ease using intuition. It is impossible to describe a 'technique' for using intuition. The only way to learn it is to listen. Ferrucci (1982) goes on to say:

We can increase our intuitive capacity if we will acknowledge the possibility of our receiving intuitions, recognize their value, cherish them when they come, and finally, learn to *trust* them.

Helpers who use intuition 'naturally' will not have analysed too much what it is that they use, or why. When they recognize an insight or a hunch, they use it as their 'sixth' sense. But those to whom it does not come naturally should not contrive it. Clients spot any incongruence as quick as lightning!

Many a time, an intuition or a hunch can summarize a helping situation.

Sensation (i.e. sense perception) tells you that something exists; *thinking* tells you what it is; *feeling* tells you whether it is agreeable or not; and *intuition* tells you whence it comes and where it is going. (Jung, 1964)

Interpretation   Intuition can at times appear to be interpretation. When using these skills in helping the client to gain new perspectives towards a goal, you need to be aware of two types of interpretation. The first type gives the client an interpretation of a situation so that an understanding of the self in relation to it can be gained.

The following conversation took place in a radiotherapy ward:

Patient: I'm slightly disappointed that the treatment isn't going to finish in three weeks but in four weeks, but I think I'm just looking at the need now and accept that.

Nurse: There is a book which points out some steps people who are seriously ill go through. One is anger: why me?

Patient: Oh goodness, yes!

Nurse: One is bargaining: if I am good now, maybe God will be good to me.

Patient: Yes (laughs).

Nurse: One is depression and this is qualified somewhat. But I am using these stages for your situation here.

Patient: Yes, go on.

Nurse: One day you'll be angry, the next day you'll be bargaining, the next day you'll be happy.

Patient: Absolutely, I had just that. My weekend consisted more or less of incredible oscillations of that nature, I went through that series, absolutely.

This kind of interpretation helped the patient to see that his disappointments and reactions to them were quite normal and that he was not 'going mad' because one moment he felt this, and another the opposite. It helped him to see himself, his disease and his treatment in perspective.

Another type of interpretation is less client centred and more helper centred:

Your problem is that you never accepted that you couldn't do that job and now everybody is suffering from your bad management.

This statement may be entirely true, but it does not help the person to do anything positive. It may well show an insecurity or impatience on the part of the helper, and therefore be hurtful and destructive. It also impinges on the rights of the person because there is no effective way of redress open.

An interpretation should be a moving-on statement, on the client's level of understanding. With empathy – being with – it is unlikely that it can go wrong.

Mind and matter

I have emphasized several times that helping is about feelings. When you want to get in touch with what a person is about, you need to get in touch with that person's feelings. But to help the person to become 'complete' and more able to function holistically, you need also to enable the thinking aspects. Setting goals is also an intellectual function. It is the time when all the various skills combine in an effort to look forward.

This may make counselling sound like a heavy and long process, which it may be, particularly perhaps with some psychiatric patients, and in developmental counselling. But it can also be easy and quick for more short-term and crisis work.

To have to think now of formulating goals should focus the attention, mobilize energy, increase persistence, and motivate the person to search for strategies (Egan, 1986).

Setting goals   How then are goals set? As a helper that may now be the appropriate question.

If the whole of the helping process has been geared towards a goal, and therefore change, that goal and that change need to be expressed in terms that are specific, and can be seen. The question here is, how are you going to do it?

Egan (1986) writes that the first point about goals is that they should be 'stated in terms of outcomes rather than behaviours leading to outcomes'. In other words, the client has first of all to believe that the goal is worthwhile, and then see it almost as already a reality. The principle of setting objectives for any task can be applied here. For example:

After reading this the helper will use counselling skills effectively at work.
When I leave hospital I will have practised looking at my wound.
In a year's time from now I will have written the first essay in my degree course. (The mother of Christopher.)

A goal has to be specific. On the whole it is not enough to say 'I must spend more time with the children'. This is a good intention, and may be the result of a deep insight. But it is not specific enough. You may need to help your client to make an intention into a detailed and distinctive goal:

| I will spend two evenings a week with the children.

When a goal is clear and specific in this way it can be measured or evaluated. At the end of the week the person can look back and see if indeed two evenings *were* spent with the children. If it wasn't possible, the reason can be established. Was it due to outside influences beyond control, or was it again work – the problem – which got in the way? If it was, was the goal realistic?

Client: I want to be with my children but I also love my work.
Helper: Which do you really love more?
Client: Work fulfils me in a way that home doesn't.
Helper: So you stay on at work and don't get home when they expect you.
Client: Work never finishes in a hospital, you know that too, and I feel needed there . . ..
Helper: How realistic then is it for you to have two evenings at home?
Client: I should be able to fit it in.
Helper: You *should*
Client: I also *want* to.
Helper: And *can* you?
Client: I could if I tried. I'll give it another go. No, wait a minute: two evenings one week, one evening the other week. That will give me a bit more leeway and will allow me to try it out more.

Revising a goal is not necessarily a step backwards. It may be a more realistic step forward. In this case the client himself had the idea of a 'compromise' with himself. This shows the self-responsibility, refusal to buckle, sense of direction, versatility and ability to transcend self-interest (mentioned on p. 96) which may ultimately be more important than keeping to a predetermined plan.

Some people only learn by their mistakes, and to let them make mistakes can be important. As helpers we are not there to punish clients, but to lead them to live more comfortably and effectively with their personal resources. It is often more advantageous to go through a failure with a person than to impose a goal which is not wholly owned. There are risks involved in doing this, and they may have to be weighed up by both helper and client. A programme which is not in keeping with the client's values may, however, be more destructive than constructive.

Finally, a goal should have some relation to time. The client above could try out his new schedule for being at home for a set period, say three months. Any such limit allows for the possibility of change.

A moral contract

When a client and helper have worked together on a problem, it is often helpful for them to share the outcome. Any evaluation is useful, but particularly one where two people were closely involved.

For a person to admit to a difficulty in front of another can sometimes be very significant. Something 'unmentionable' spelled out is a form of getting rid of it. Talking about it is cleansing. It is also a kind of commitment to carry out what has been talked about. The issue is now not any longer only in the mind of one person; it is shared. Two people are now involved. There is therefore a moral 'contract' as well as a practical one. This may sometimes have to be pointed out.

Having such a contract is more than the nuts and bolts of meeting. It is also more than simply being kind and telling the helper of the successes achieved, showing what a good client he or she is by doing what had been promised. Such a contract can be an important step for the client in becoming more truly human by being true to the self.

Many self-help agencies work on the principle of behaviourism: using rewards or punishments for goals achieved. This may occasionally apply to the helping you do with patients. But equally it may be too limiting. What matters is that helping is effective all along the line, right up to the very tip of the diamond.

Goal setting may be the time when some action takes place: something is moving. That movement follows some fairly clear lines. It is also a movement of integration and both client and helper may need unusual skills in the unique situation in which they find themselves.

11 Counselling skills: challenging

Challenging

It has been said that the whole of the counselling process is a challenge. The client seeks help because he is stuck, and to get out of that situation some attitude or behaviour has to be challenged.

To challenge someone is indeed a skill. But it is not just one specific skill. It is a question of using all the helping skills and tactics in such a way that the client is gently pushed, pulled or prodded. Any challenge is *for* the client, and only with the client's goal in mind. Challenge should be positive; it is never meant for punishing.

Challenge has something negative about it, therefore it should first of all reinforce. Challenge the strengths of a person rather than the weaknesses. Point out a person's strengths, resources and assets as they may not otherwise be recognized fully.

Any challenge should be concrete and specific. Simply to say 'you need to become more assertive' is not enough.

In a group, one person may say to another:

I like what you are saying, but I would like to hear more of it! You put yourself in the background and then others get there before you, and they don't listen to you. Sometimes it's hard to hear you because you speak so softly. But what you say is always worth hearing.

You handled that very well, but your voice was still a bit shaky and I could sense that you had to control yourself.

The manner in which a challenge is offered is very important. People are like china shops, and you can't walk into people's feelings as if you were a bull. On the other hand, you don't go in apologizing either. When the moment and the occasion is right for a challenge, do it carefully but surely:

From what you say it seems that you have not looked at this aspect very carefully. Perhaps it isn't easy, but should you give it some thought now?

This is a gentle way of offering a challenge. It is also true, but perhaps sometimes not taken seriously enough by counsellors, that people are robust and can take a challenge. They often ask for it; they need it – always with the aim of seeing the way forward.

When there is a reason to challenge, your professional integrity demands that you do it. Otherwise the client may not be able to develop with your help, but may remain in the morass, and perhaps even sink further into it.

One way of using challenging as a skill is with the 'sandwich technique', as with the example of the group above. First you give praise or reinforcement: one slice of bread. Then you give the challenge: the important filling. Then you give more reinforcement or praise: the other slice of bread.

Patient: I only smoked ten cigarettes all last week, but I've already had ten this week, and it's only Monday.

Nurse: You did really well last week, congratulations! Tell me why you think you have already had too many this week.

Patient: (describes in detail)

Nurse: Last week you were very enthusiastic and it was easy. This week your friends are on holiday and they visit you and while they smoke, you smoke with them. It's difficult to refuse them! Perhaps you need to look more closely at the way you say 'no' to your friends. But the fact that you managed to keep to your goal last week is the first step in the right direction.

Egan (1986) suggests that helpers actually have to earn the right to challenge. They should not challenge others unless they challenge themselves in the way they live and develop physically, intellectually, socially and emotionally. Unless they also develop professionally, the insights they may have gained into themselves will become obsolete. When clients see that their helpers are challengeable they may accept challenge from them more easily.

Blockages to change

What do you challenge? What is it in the helping process that needs to be challenged?

Sometimes clients and their attitudes or behaviours are like flies on a window. They buzz around, making a great deal of noise, expending vast amounts of energy, acting as if the window would thereby go away, when only a few inches away a window is open and they could fly through it. But that behaviour, and in the case of humans also that attitude, prevents them from moving even just a very short distance. The skill here is to challenge the behaviours or attitudes which block a movement forward. Essentially you challenge the blind spots in the person's vision of the future.

Dan, a 45-year-old father of two teenage sons, had a relapse of his multiple sclerosis. The health visitor called regularly. His wife had told him that she would leave him for another man in ten days but would still come back regularly 'to visit the boys'. Dan was devastated.

Patient: I hate her for this, and yet I can't stop my love for her either after all this time.

Nurse: It must be very confusing to have her still here and yet to know that she also belongs somewhere else.

Patient: I want her to feel that this is still her home and that she can come back any time.

Nurse: That's very generous and surely the right thing to do.

Later in the conversation

Patient: We've more or less settled things financially, so when she goes all I will do then is to take the house-key off her.

Nurse: You said earlier that you would do everything to make her still feel at home here. Now you say you'll take the key off her. That sounds contradictory to me.

Patient: Goodness, I never thought of it in this way.

Months later, the fact that Dan had been generous and had let her keep the key, and she had access to the house, seemed to be the element which brought them together again in a new way.

The blockages to change are the inconsistencies in people's lives: inconsistencies between what they say and do; what they think they do and really do; who they imagine themselves to be and really are. This last is particularly often evident in people who think they are assertive, whereas in fact they are either manipulative or destructive.

Some people adopt defence mechanisms to avoid dealing with difficulties. This can show itself in adopting a helpless or hopeless attitude. Particularly in patients with serious illness, the attitude can become one of having no control over the situation, or that a negative outcome of a prognosis is experienced as if it had already come about (Moorey and Greer, 1989).

Another feature of blockages to change are negative thoughts (see p. 84).

Two nurses reminiscing about their training days:

A: Isn't it funny how one seems to remember only the demeaning things.
B: That's what *you* remember.
A: But . . ..
B: I remember the crises, and they weren't necessarily 'bad'.
A: I never thought of it like that.

Nelson-Jones (1988) mentions irrational beliefs as blockages and blind spots. A 'must' rules.

I must be treated in the way I tell them to.
I must get through this. (See p. 82.)

Such a belief sets up an inner rule which leads to irrational consequences.

Resistance and avoidance

Most of us will at some stage have said that, when a patient begins to resist care or treatment, he is getting better.

Resistance and avoidance are two particular types of blind spots and therefore merit particular attention.

As with all such mechanisms, there is a reason why a person is resistant, in this context resistant to help offered. A person may be a 'professional resister', rebelling against any system; or think that needing help is admitting defeat; or feel the need for personal power and express it by resisting someone considered to be more powerful.

Avoidance is similar to reluctance. Egan (1982) says that 'avoidance behaviour is one of the principal mechanisms contributing to the psychopathology of the average'. People stay in the morass of being average because they avoid confronting themselves and their behaviours.

Avoidance patterns are learnt from early childhood (see p. 23). We consciously steer clear of difficult situations by avoiding them. When we sense something difficult coming our way, we get on guard.

For example, some people cannot take criticism, so if they sense that something of that nature may be going on, they change the subject. Two people who tend to disagree with each other about a certain issue ultimately learn not to talk about that issue. In this way each avoids an uncomfortable situation. Jung (1933) noted that

> Every one of us gladly turns away from his problems; if possible, they must not be mentioned, or better still, their existence is denied. We wish to make our lives simple, certain and smooth – and for that reason problems are taboo.

One way of avoiding what is happening is to talk about it in the third person.

> The light is at the end of the tunnel somewhere and one can't yet see it get bigger. In the early stages of treatment one seems to be able to cope, and then the light seems to get smaller, and then one imagines things.

Such polite talk is often a way of avoiding looking at what is going on. Yet the problem is not in 'one', but in 'me'. Looking at 'me' is direct, and disturbing. In looking at myself, I may not like what I see, therefore I avoid it.

All blockages to growth are difficult to deal with. The most helpful way may be to treat them positively and work with them, rather than against them. They are in themselves negative and often destructive, so it is easy to give in to them, but that simply feeds them.

Challenging blind spots and other discrepancies is necessary for the release of energy for more appropriate action. In Egan's (1986) words this would amount to taking stock of the present scenario, going on to the preferred scenario ('What would your world look like if it were a little better?') and finally to action.

Confronting with reality

What is actually happening when some blind spot is challenged is that the person can see the reality of the world as it is at that point, whereas before it was distorted by behaviours and rules which had become the inner driving force.

Confronting someone with reality in a helping relationship is not a putting down.

Through confrontation we challenge the discrepancies, the distortions, the games, the unwillingness to understand, the unproductive behaviours that plague our interpersonal lives. (Egan, 1977)

A very simple and perhaps even obvious example of the discrepancies which are often all too evident is shown in this extract from a conversation.

Patient: No really, I'm fine.

Nurse: You are progressing as far as your health is concerned, but the way you look, and you are sitting so tightly in the corner of your chair, makes me think that you have a lot of pain inside yourself.

Patient: (loosening herself and after a long moment) I do have pain . . . It's the anniversary of my mother's death, and she had cancer too.

The following is from a personal journal of a nurse:

At first he talked and talked, and I listened, and in fact I would not have been able to get a word in edgeways. I was aware that I was listening without being reflective, and so, little by little, I started to reflect some of the things back to him in a digested way. I felt I had to feed him a bit of the reality of what is happening to other patients with his sort of condition. I said that when he was admitted his behaviour was very much that of letting us know that here comes A. He had to prove to us that he was still himself, that he was normal, and that he was going to kick against anything that was in any way abnormal. I felt that having said that, this was like a reassurance to him that he is in fact normal, that he has progressed since then, that we had accepted him as he was then, and as he is now, and also that we care about him. I felt that by giving him little bits of himself at a time, and by reflecting back what he had just given me in the way of information, I was able to confront him with the reality appropriate to him.

The four questions: What is happening? What is the meaning of it? What is your goal? What are you doing about it? may very well highlight some discrepancies and reveal the reality relevant to that person's life, and help to acknowledge and adopt it for a more satisfying life-style.

Immediacy

The skill of immediacy is another of the ways of challenging in helping. Egan (1977) calls this the skill of 'you–me talk', as it is used particularly for looking at the relationship between helper and client. Perhaps not surprisingly, clients are often not fully aware of how they affect other people. Most difficulties in anybody's life are those of relationships. It is therefore quite likely that the difficulties clients have with their relationships generally are also mirrored in this relationship with you now. Using the skill of immediacy may be a very powerful way of introducing this particular reality (Woolfe, 1989).

The following is a patient talking to the breast-care nurse after a mastectomy. It may almost follow the story on p. 84, and may indicate how difficult, yet important, it is for patients and clients to talk about sexual matters.

Patient: We've never had a marvellous sex life, but just now when I most need to feel I am still a woman he (her husband) is now totally impotent.

Nurse: You mentioned having to feel like a woman before; what does this actually mean to you?

Patient: I think you are not taking me seriously. I am asking you to help me with his impotence.

Nurse: Can I stop here for a moment and actually look at what is going on between us two.

Patient: Well, go on then.

Nurse: As I just said, you mentioned several times having to feel like a woman, and each time I asked you to think about it you switched the conversation away from you. I feel that you are asking for something but then refuse it when it is offered. I am actually feeling impotent to help you – or perhaps more strongly, I feel made impotent.

Patient: Are you saying that I am making my husband impotent?

Nurse: Not exactly. What I am saying is that our relationship here may very well mirror something that is going on at home.

Patient: I don't quite follow you.

Nurse: I feel that your relationship with your husband may have some element in it which is similar to your relationship with me. You may be asking something of him but when he tries to give it to you, you don't accept it.

Patient: But you are not my husband.

Nurse: No, but I am picking up a similar way of behaving.

Patient: What am I asking from him then?

Nurse: You are asking from him how to be a woman.

Patient: And he doesn't give it to me by being impotent.

Nurse: You are asking me too, how can you be a woman?

Patient: Yes?

Nurse: How can you be a woman?

Patient: Well, how?

Nurse: Stay with that question for a while.

Patient: I don't know if I like it now.

Nurse: I expect that for you 'being a woman' is something far more important than the words might convey. I am pushing you now to perhaps look at that side of it, and perhaps your husband is pushing you in the same way to look at yourself, because you actually ask for it. What do you feel when I push you in this way?

Patient: Go away! It's rather hot!

Nurse: How does that tie in with your husband's 'going away'?

Sometimes clients think that if you can tell them what a third person should do, or say, the situation would improve. You cannot 'counsel' a third person, or effect a change in that person. You cannot even change the client. You can *help* the client to change himself, and the client can then influence the relationship with that third person in the way which is most appropriate. The relationship between helper and client therefore becomes a model, and a place for trying out new behaviours. In what way is the relationship between helper and client different from the problematic one? What does this one have which the other doesn't? What is better here than there?

Egan (1977) says that, like other relationship skills, immediacy has three parts:

1. Awareness.
2. Communication know-how.
3. Assertiveness or 'guts'.

In the example above these are evident in the fact that the helper also became aware of a sense of impotence in her: she could not function adequately. The communication know-how was shown in that she knew when to intervene and in a way which the client could understand. The client showed a great deal of resistance to understanding, but that is the nature of blind spots and blockages. The assertiveness of the helper was then shown in the way in which she stuck with her intervention and did not retaliate or answer in an aggressive way.

Overcoming blocks

Any challenge to blockages and blind spots is for the client's greater sense of well-being and more satisfying life. The operative words at this stage must therefore surely be self-responsibility, self help skills, **and empowerment**.

All the help you give to any person is to empower that person. Someone who has power, real, authentic power, is likely to use it in a responsible way. Such a person will use their power mainly to empower others. The people who either do not have power, or only think they have it, use power in ways which are often dangerous: by manipulating or with aggression. Therefore, to help someone to use their own power more adequately and fully is to liberate them from the bondages of deficiencies and inadequacies.

One of the most effective ways of overcoming blocks is by imagination (see p. 97). How would the world be if it were a little different? This question so often holds the key to more adequate living. The point of helping and counselling is that it should be self-perpetuating: once the client has found the key, it is handed on to others, like a relay. Key questions therefore become the self-help tools which empower ever more people.

Another very useful way of dealing with blocks is by visualization. This has been widely used by Simonton et al. (1978) with patients who have cancer. Gawain (1978) has made visualization much more widely applicable. She calls the basic steps in creative visualization:

1. Setting your goal.
2. Creating a clear idea of picture.
3. Focusing on it often.
4. Giving it positive energy.

These steps seem remarkably similar to the basic helping models and principles. Visualizing better relationships, as an example, can also be a way of finding alternatives to present blocks. The skills lie with the client; the helper may only have to be the 'midwife' in suggesting the technique in the first place, but ultimately it is the client who has to do it.

This chapter concludes the discussion of the main elements of helping people by counselling.

The examples given are as near 'perfect' as possible. The whole thing looks easy on paper. Theories are wonderful things but life is neither perfect, easy, nor wonderful. You will not meet the same examples. It would be so good to 'have the answer' but there is no answer, or at least not an easy one.

The more you can forget about theories, and the right thing to say, the better. The more you can be yourself, the better. But that takes courage. When you can forget about skills and the role you have, and become you, the more you are enabling the other person to do likewise, and that is what it is all about.

12 Specific issues

Because the nature of counselling and helping is interpersonal, a range of issues surrounding relationships inevitably gets connected with it. Some of the issues mentioned in this chapter are more important for some people than others. Depending on the setting and type of helping, some are present and some are not. Not to draw attention to them would be an omission; yet to mention them in a setting for nurses could give the impression that counselling is therapy, which generally it is not. Perhaps, as with most other issues in helping and counselling, awareness of these various issues is the main necessity.

Opportunities for counselling

The daily life of a nurse is full of opportunities for helping in a counselling manner. What matters is the way in which you react to and deal with each opportunity.

Your role is first of all that of nurse, and your setting is that of sickrooms, wards, clinics, and associated places.

When you are bathing patients they are *physically* exposed. The step towards exposing themselves *emotionally* is not great. Confidences are made and problems aired, which, perhaps like the hurting body part, can only be dealt with behind screens or when there is total attention.

It is at these times that the patients will come out with

My husband and I never talk about dying.
I had never said this to anybody, but . . . .
How do you think I am getting on?
That patient over there worries me. I've never seen anybody so ill.
What if I can't walk any more?

All these subtle questions can have a straightforward

practical answer. But the setting in which they are asked probably means that that is not what they need. They need the small space of person-to-person contact and, in a way, demand that you, the nurse, 'expose' yourself too by your helping.

The situation may also be the other way round. The patient has never said anything remotely personal or which showed any self-awareness, and *you* feel that the patient has a problem which should be discussed. How do you go about it? This is far more delicate because you are imposing your values and standards on another person. All the communication skills you have are then needed. It is possible that by showing concern the patient may respond. It is possible that he may choose not you, but the least likely person in the team to confide in. What you cannot do is to make anybody talk. You cannot 'counsel' someone; you can only help them to ask for counselling, if that is what they need. Brown (1988) writes:

The comment of the mother of a 30-year-old man who died angry, in physical pain and mental torment, makes us stop and think. When one of the doctors explained how sad the team was, and felt that they had been able to help John so little, his mother said 'But he was an angry young man. He was a fighter all his life, and I'm glad you didn't change him'.

There are numerous practical problems which interfere with making the most of an opportunity: you talk with a patient and just then the telephone rings, your bleep goes, or you are called to an emergency. However much you try, you cannot really return to the patient and the subject easily. Or a patient may catch you just as you are going out of the door after a heavy day, when you have no more physical or emotional strength left. Or you go into the room of a very sick person whose hand lies on the bed begging to be held. Fear of what to say, or embarrassment may make you pretend not to notice it but instead busy yourself with all sorts of extras, like clearing out dead flowers.

Opportunities present themselves at every turn. Some you can deal with, some not. It may not matter so much when you *cannot* deal with them, for the patients will understand that. The difficulty is when you *won't* deal with them. You can't be giving all the time. When you can't, simply acknowledge your need. That in itself will be helpful.

Making a contract

It has been said that a contract is that which makes the difference between counselling and helping.

A professional counsellor will make a contract with the client which spells out clearly how often they will meet, for how long, what it costs and how and when payment should be made, and what the conditions are for cancellation.

None of this is so clearly present when counselling takes place within another framework, such as nursing or social work. Counselling is 'on the hoof' and only part of other work. The clear exception is counselling in mental health settings. Here, contracts play a large role, often as part of social skills training. People who are out of touch with social boundaries can gradually be reintroduced to living alongside other people by respecting such contracts.

But sometimes it is also possible, and necessary or desirable, to have something like a contract even in very simple settings. It may be possible to put a time limit on a request, or decide to meet again, or ask for space.

Patient: I know you are busy, but have you got a minute?
Nurse: I've got ten minutes, is that enough?

Patient: I see you are just going home, but I've been trying to catch you all day.
Nurse: How urgent is the problem? You are right, I am on my way home.
Patient: Well, it won't go away, but it can wait until tomorrow.
Nurse: I will make a point of seeing you tomorrow morning.
Patient: Thank you, that will be fine.

Nurse: It seems to me that there is plenty more there to talk about.
Patient: I've had enough for one day now.
Nurse: Would you like me to come again tomorrow?
Patient: Not tomorrow, but Saturday. I won't have any visitors then.
Nurse: That's fine, I'm working late on Saturday. It's a deal.

These are some possible contracts. The important thing is that they are kept. If you have ten minutes to give to a person, give the ten minutes wholly, not thinking of all the other things you could be doing instead. If you say ten minutes, given ten, not eight or twenty minutes.

If you do set time aside to talk with a patient, perhaps tell a colleague that you don't want to be disturbed.

Above all, if possible never make assumptions: 'Oh, I know what my client wants anyway'. This time the client may want something different. The person who wants a 'word' with you may need many such words, and immediately; or this may simply be the only perceived way of asking you for something that may take just a sentence to answer. Check it out. Can it wait for your convenience or would it add to your client's pain and yours if you didn't deal with it at once?

Endings and detachment

All of us know the situation in which the most important thing in a conversation was said as the person was getting up from the chair, or standing in the doorway. Ending a counselling session or process is as difficult and as important as beginning one.

Most of the counselling situations in nursing are short. Notable exceptions are those in mental health, the care of the elderly, and in community nursing. In these settings, where relationships are long term, the ending may have to be prepared for and worked on. The severing of a long and perhaps close personal tie may be like a death. For many patients this may be repeating a process which they have already gone through in relation to their own illness. If an important person in their life now leaves as well, this may evoke the old pain. Feelings of rejection by and hostility towards the helper may be quite strong, and to some extent legitimate.

In more short-term situations there are other difficulties. Patients may on occasion feel ashamed that they might have uncovered more about themselves than they were initially prepared for. Or they may wonder why they 'burdened that young girl' with their story in the first place. A simple statement that it was you who encouraged them to do so may be reassuring. It can also help to say to a patient at the end that you are aware that this sort of talking may have made him uncomfortable. Confirmation that anything said between helper and client is confidental may also be helpful at the moment of ending.

People who say the most important thing when the time is up have a reason for doing it in this way. They may not have trusted themselves to talk about it before, or may have wanted to test the helper out first to see if the helper could be trusted. It may be important at such a time to acknowledge that you have heard the throw-away remark, but that the time is now up. To indicate when you will be available again may not only be polite, but may encourage a sense of security and continuity.

It may sometimes be helpful in counselling to state shortly before the end that there are only so many minutes left. This can help clients to get their priorities in order at that moment. Flexibility and firmness have to be combined in endings, as do genuine care and genuine challenge.

In the analogy of the victim in the ditch (see Chapter 9), both helper and client are eventually on the road, on firm ground, and each needs to go his own way. The purpose of helping is to let the client find his own road, and for him to be pleased to take it.

The person who teaches another to ride a bicycle, or to swim, will sooner or later have to give him a push and then let go. Perhaps the difference between sympathy and empathy is that push. You say to the client, you *are* yourself, now *be* yourself.

One reason for supervision (see Chapter 2) is that a helper sometimes has

a blind spot about endings (and) he may deny how important people are to him, and he to them; or he may have a different problem, that of being able to let people go. (Jacobs, 1982)

It may be as difficult for the helper to let go as it is for the client. The awareness (What is happening?) and the point (What is the meaning of it?) can lead to a redefinition (What is the goal?) by being self-responsible and skilled (What am I going to do about it?).

Transference and counter-transference

Transference is something which can happen without being acknowledged by either side and it is easily disguised. It is the shifting of an affect from one person to another, or from one idea to another, especially the transfer by the patient to the analyst of emotional tones, of either affection or hostility, based on unconscious identification. (Olson-Dorland, 1969)

Transference is particularly evident in psychoanalysis. There it 'is part of the planned process of bringing unconscious material into consciousness' (Altschul and

Sinclair, 1981). Counselling is less geared to deliberately calling up unconscious material, therefore transference is less of a specific tool in this type of helping. Nevertheless, transference is very often present.

Patients in hospital sometimes behave as if they were in love with nurses when, in fact, they invest in the nurse the love which they feel for their mother.
Relatives may be afraid to ask doctors for their opinion and may treat doctors with the deference which might have been appropriate for their own fathers. Parents often transfer to their children's teacher the mixture of fear and respect they formerly had for their own headmaster. Nurses may find that their attitude towards the sister or nursing officer is irrational and represents a transference of feelings from their own family experience. (Altschul and Sinclair, 1981)

Some of these feelings are misplaced and irrational, but because of their very existence they are important and may throw light on other feelings or behaviours. Clients use us (and we use others) to act out relationships with other significant people in their (or our) lives.
Miller (1981) says that transference is

essentially a defence mechanism, designed to protect ourselves and preserve our security. Knowing ourselves may be threatening, and the more threatening it is, the more likely a person is to project.

A transference, or projection, is always about a feeling, usually an unfinished feeling from the past, and often not related clearly to what is going on now. However, if such feelings can be faced and used, then they can become integral parts of the helping process and lead the patient or client to own the past and the present with a view to being a more whole and 'potent' person in the future.
Transference means that a patient projects a feeling on to you; in countertransference you then project back to the client your own unacknowledged feelings. Lefébure (1985) quotes Audrey Hepburn from the film *Funny Face* where she played the part of a woman to whom a philosopher makes amorous advances and she said: 'I thought you were a philosopher, you're just a man'. If you let yourself act in the role in which you are cast by the client, then you countertransfer. But when you treat the patient (the philosopher) as a *man*, not as the lover

he would like himself to be, then you can help him; otherwise you are locked into a no-win situation.

Involvement

'Don't get involved!' is a cry which is often heard in nursing; or 'She got over-involved' is whispered with an air of 'She should have known better'. It is precisely the workings of transference and countertransference which are revealed here. Because they are irrational, unconscious defence mechanisms, they are not understood and thus feared. The easiest way to deal with them is therefore not to allow them into the light. Sadly, that is destructive, more than dealing with the feelings and projections themselves.

I have argued in this book that to help anybody emotionally, you need to deal with their feelings. It is the feelings which have priority in helping. But feelings need empathy to be useful. Without empathy, feelings run away with us, overpower us and frighten us. With empathy, feelings become our friends and helpers. Now empathy is a way of being: being with people and their feelings. It is also a way of being with ourselves and our feelings. This means that we are *already* 'involved'. The way to behave appropriately is therefore to be 'involved' appropriately. To be aware: aware of what is going on; aware of pitfalls and blind spots; aware of fears and shortcomings. But just as individual clients are unable to extricate themselves from a difficult situation, so we, the helpers, also need support, in the form of supervision.

To say 'Don't get involved' is defeating. Empathy goes down or alongside the 'involved' person, finds out what the problem is, and with one foot on the firm ground introduces different perspectives and thus enables and empowers the person to go on his or her own way again.

Involvement usually points to a countertransference situation. Lefébure (1985) calls countertransference a 'trap'; and being a trap, there is no way out of it alone. But with the companionship of empathy it can be seen again for what it is, acknowledged, and changed.

Dependence on clients

A few words are needed to elaborate on the helper's need to be needed.

Helpers don't only have needs to be helped; they have deep needs to be needed. There is nothing wrong in that. It only becomes dangerous when this need is misused.

If you were asked why you went into nursing, you will probably answer that it was because you wanted to help people. If you were further asked why you wanted to help people, you might not be able to give a very clear answer; it might perhaps be something on the lines of wanting to care for people less fortunate.

When you are helping people to deal with an important aspect of their lives, you are likely to ask them for the (or a) meaning in their lives. This may uncover a number of unknown elements.

In Chapter 11 I made the point that helpers need to be willing to be challenged, and therefore I am asking here, what is your meaning in life? You can only ask others what you can also ask yourself. You can only teach others what you also know yourself. I will go further and say, we can only do to others what we also do to ourselves. We love others only when we love ourselves. We are nurses to others only when we know how to be nurses to ourselves. We only hurt others because we also hurt ourselves. We only need others because we are needy in ourselves.

Human nature is such that we *do* need each other for living. But to *use* others to boost ourselves is unhelpful for both parties; in that case, neither side can grow. When you come to the awareness, and act on it, that you walk side by side on the road of life, not carried on each other's backs, then you set each other free.

When you acknowledge your needs then they become tools for you to work with, rather than luggage which you demand others to carry for you. When you allow yourself to acknowledge your needs, then you become free to help. Then your needs will be met by all those you help; but that is incidental. It does not happen if you ask your clients to fulfil your needs, thus keeping them dependent on you.

This chapter highlights once again the various and often hidden agendas that each person has. As a helper you have just as many as your clients have. All of these issues are not either right or wrong. They simply *are*. The way you *are* with them is what matters.

One of the comments about counselling sometimes made by teachers and tutors is that it is impossible to know what is 'their' and what is 'your' (my) business.

Looking at this issue in the light of awareness, and perhaps transference and countertransference, and how they are set up and maintained, may help to make the distinction and lessen the burden or confusion.

13 Specific situations

It is impossible to say that one type of nurse or another is more vulnerable; that this situation or that is more difficult. Any situation or problem can be easy or difficult, depending on any number of factors. What is easy for one person is difficult for another. The difference probably 'only' lies in the experience. Since counsellors are not born, but made, no situation should ever be beyond help, even if only 'beginner's help'.

Sometimes you will be faced with completely unexpected situations or remarks and you are inevitably surprised. Nursing will already have helped you to develop a certain unshockability. It is definitely an advantage to have that, together with a non-judgemental attitude and perhaps an ability to see the funny side of things occasionally.

Patients with mental handicaps

People who are mentally handicapped have similar problems to other people. The difficulties are not just to do with their handicap; those who have been in hospitals for a long time inevitably have problems concerned with institutionalization.

Mentally handicapped people are, perhaps more than other people, used to having decisions made for them, even having a sentence finished for them. Taking responsibility for themselves is therefore something which they may neither understand nor be willing to have.

Counselling as such is often to do with major decisions in their lives, such as moving from an institution to a hostel, or into the community. It may be very difficult for people with a mental handicap to understand what this involves for them, or what they are expected to do.

Riley (1983) found that most of her difficulties were 'pitching what you say at the right level so that you are both talking about the same thing'. Some things have to be stated very simply, and be repeated often. It may also be necessary to bear in mind that some handicapped people have unusual facial expressions, so it may be difficult to gauge if what has been said 'got through', and if the response will be as expected. There may be no outward sign of change in mood, and that may be difficult for the counsellor.

Because some people have difficulty expressing feelings does not mean to say that they do not have any. Helping mentally handicapped people express their feelings may help them to bring meaning and wholeness into their lives; but perhaps not as quickly as for other people. Using counselling skills correctly is therefore even more important for this group of people.

Counselling children

Young children have a different understanding and experience of the world from adults. Counselling in adult terms is therefore not relevant to small children. What matters is that they are heard and responded to at the appropriate level and in the appropriate manner.

It should be realized that very ill children often have an intuitive knowledge about death and dying. Explanations should be given in simple words and metaphors which they can understand, such as making comparisons with pets who have died.

More taxing for nurses is the help which parents need. It is they who bear a heavy burden with sick children. Despite what they may think, their children are often very astute at realizing when parents are worried or fearful. When the parents feel at ease, the child becomes at ease. Helping and counselling the parents may therefore be the priority.

Siblings tend to be the forgotten party in these situations. The parents have to care for the sick child, and siblings are left to cope. Although they may not have much contact with hospital nursing staff, the situation in the community is quite different. Here, a nurse may get to know the family situation well and find it particularly appropriate to consider the family as a whole when offering help.

**The
'problem'
patient**

There will always be people with whom you have difficulty developing a fruitful relationship. You try to help, but they refuse help. You try to cajole, and they don't want to know. You try to humour them, and they think you don't take them seriously.

Perhaps the most difficult patients are those who ask for your help but reject it. They do this to everybody else: each nurse will hear the story, and it is normally a long one. Day after day they drain you of your energy. What is more, having done the round of all the possible people, they are then in a position to play one person off against another. 'Do you know what the physio suggested? She said I should lose weight! What an effrontery!' Because of a respect for confidentiality, you are caught in a web of intrigue. The patient wants help, but is not able to use the help offered.

Such patients are themselves caught in a world of fantasy and make-believe. They think that they are victims and need to be rescued. And nurses, like most health care workers, have a strong sense of rescuing, and they are seduced.

The story of the man in the ditch (see Chapter 9) shows quite clearly that he was not rescued, but helped to stand on his own feet, and so could walk away from the spot under his own steam. People who take on the role of victim have been hurt somewhere in life, but that behaviour is now not relevant any more and should if possible be challenged. Moreover, what they present as a problem is unlikely to be the real problem, which they cannot talk about because, if they did, they would expose a side of themselves which is weak, helpless and quite inadequate. So they play the game of deception.

Patient: Nurse, will you help me sort this out?
Nurse: I'll try.
Patient: I spoke to Nurse J. yesterday, but she was so rude that I don't want to speak to her any more.

The trap here is to be shocked by Nurse J's remark and so get away from the problem.

Nurse: How can I help you?
Patient: Well, you said I could go home next week, but you see I can't use that arm at all well, and how can I look after myself with one useless arm and the other not strong enough?
Nurse: We've talked about that several times already and there all sorts of possibilities.

Patient: But you don't understand! I simply have no-one to help me.

Another trap. you don't understand me. The nurse is made to feel that she is no good, or should defend herself.

Nurse: I'm beginning to feel that you are afraid of something at home. You've lived alone so long.

Patient: You nurses are all the same. You never believe what anybody says and read things into situations which you don't know anything about.

The patient becomes defensive. This probably proves that the nurse is on to something 'real'.

Nurse: Are you afraid of something at home?
Patient: Of course not, what makes you think that?
Nurse: I just thought I could detect a note of fear in your voice.
Patient: I'm all right.
Nurse: I just have a hunch that something is not all right.
Patient: I don't have a problem at home.
Nurse: Is the problem somewhere else?
Patient: You are persistent, aren't you?

This may mean: leave me alone. Or it may mean: you are right, go on.

Nurse: I am, but tell me if I'm not right.
Patient: Well . . ..
Nurse: What is it, can you tell me?
Patient: It's a long story, but I just hate that flat.
Nurse: Go on.

This story (the patient eventually revealed that she hated her flat because her husband had died there; she felt that she had killed him and the memory constantly haunted her) shows that by not giving in to the many traps laid, but by (1) concentrating on the patient and her feelings, and (2) following her intuition, the nurse got to a point where something could be 'moved'. The patient's own defensive mechanism kept her locked into a situation which was increasingly unbearable and unproductive, not to mention the undesirability of keeping her in care and dependent when she could be independent. In this case the nurse referred the patient to a social worker who helped her with her long-term emotional problem as well as with housing.

Relatives

Sometimes the problem is not the patient, but the family. At the bedside of the patient are now acted out all manner of family dynamics which perhaps were never dealt with before.

Those who were formerly independent and dominant will have become dependent, and vice versa. The role of carer and cared-for will have been reversed. It is easy to underestimate the immense process of adjustment involved in this change. Children find it difficult to come to terms with the responsibilities involved, and parents find it difficult to relinquish them. (Scrutton, 1989)

So you get into situations of 'Don't tell him, he couldn't cope', or 'I'm the spokesperson for the family', but the other members tell you that they don't trust him. As the nurse, you are inevitably 'pig-in-the-middle', either trying to keep the parties together or apart.

It is an understatement to say that this is not easy. As a nurse you have your own feelings and values to consider, and your own, the patient's and the family's integrity to maintain.

Like the patient, the family may accept or reject your help. Like the patient, you can only offer help but not make them take it. You cannot 'counsel' them if they are not willing to be counselled.

Depending on how long the patient remains in your care, you may be able to loosen some knots which may be preventing free-flowing relationships. You may be able to present a different point of view from the one held by the family and enable them to take it on board safely. You may be able to use your position in the middle as a real go-between and help to heal old rifts. You may be able to place anger and resentments where they properly belong (in the past) by helping both sides to see what they are doing to each other.

Helping and counselling members of the family is the same as helping and counselling patients. The only thing to keep in mind, if you are helping both sides, is that their respective confidences have to be kept separate unless you have permission from one side or the other to pass on anything relevant.

Families often rely on nurses as much as do the patients themselves, and it can be rewarding to leave a whole family unit in a better state than when it first came into your care.

Dying and death

The care of dying people has received a great deal of attention in recent years, and more and more nurses, not only those in hospices, feel increasingly comfortable with it. Nevertheless, most nurses still fear the outright question 'Am I dying?', although experience shows that it is seldom asked in this way.

> Do you think I'm really getting better?
> I know it will soon be my turn.
> It's a funny thing, dying. I can understand now why people will try every treatment they can get.

Kübler-Ross (1970) was one of the first people who classified the process of dying into stages. Since then, these stages have been adapted (Speck, 1978) and widened (Charles-Edwards, 1983). The essential elements of the process are: denial, anger, fear and resolution. It is important to realize that here, too, the stages can all be muddled up, and a patient who one day is angry, may the next day be accepting the situation, and the third day be paralysed with fear. Brown (1988) lists the principles of help and support given to people who are dying as: (1) never tell a lie; (2) never take away all hope; (3) listen well.

Brown gives a good example of how these principles have been put into action.

> Mrs Todd was a 46-year-old patient with a glioma. One new development in the day before the following conversation was the onset of marked weakness in her right leg. The nurse had taken Mrs Todd her night-time medication, and had listened while Mrs Todd told her some of the day's events, and of her husband's and children's visits that evening. As the nurse turned to go, Mrs Todd called her back.

Patient: 'Nurse!'
The nurse turned and took the few steps back toward the bed.
Patient: 'Do you think I might die suddenly in the night?'

A categoric 'No' would have been certainly unhelpful and possibly untrue. Mrs Todd could have a haemorrhage into the tumour, or indeed, she could have a heart attack. Patients with cancer are not immune from these, but neither was there a high degree of likelihood, and to have mentioned them would have served no useful purpose.

Nurse: 'I think that is highly unlikely, Mrs. Todd'.

The temptation was to hurry back to the medicine trolley, but there were likely to be more worries behind Mrs Todd's question. She would probably only go on if she felt the nurse had time. This was communicated much more clearly non-verbally, than it could have been verbally. Staying, sitting, and sharing concerned attention, helped Mrs Todd to go on to ask about another patient in the ward.

Patient: 'But Mrs Green over there has been getting up much less lately, and today she's been in bed all day, and has hardly stirred.'

Nurse: 'Yes, she has been getting gradually more tired and sleepy over the past few days'.

Patient: 'Do you think that will happen to me?'

Nurse: 'Yes, I think it probably will when the time comes, though not just yet'.

Patient: 'What do the nurses do when they pull the curtains round her bed every so often?'

Nurse: 'Well the nurses move Mrs Green's position so that she does not become sore. If you look next time the nurses have been to her, you'll find she is facing the opposite way. They also moisten her mouth to keep it comfortable, now that she cannot drink.'

Patient: 'And her husband? He has been sitting there all day – my husband won't be able to do that. He can't bear being here, and doesn't stay very long. What will the nurses think of him?'

Nurse: 'It is important for relatives to do what feels right and comfortable for them. We will try to help him to do that. His way may be different, but not better or worse.'

Patient: 'And that bag – will I have one of those? Now my leg is weaker, I have to have a commode by the bed, but what if I can't make it out of bed? I couldn't bear to make a mess.'

Nurse: 'Yes, if that should happen we will be able to use a catheter to drain the urine as we have with Mrs Green.'

Patient: 'I have been so worried today, not knowing what was happening to Mrs Green; and yet she seems comfortable and peaceful, and still cared for. But it helps to know what's happening. Thank you. You must get on now, and I'll get to sleep.'

The next morning, Mrs Todd told one of the doctors that since she had been ill, she had wondered what dying would be like. It had helped to talk about what was happening to Mrs Green.

Nurses often feel that they should answer a straight 'Am I dying?' with a straight 'Yes' or 'No'. They say that *they* would like to know if they asked that question. One way of looking at this dilemma is with the help of the four questions (see Chapter 5).

1. *What is happening?* The patient will have some reason for asking that question. He or she may not be feeling well; certain investigations will have aroused suspicion; some remarks dropped were perhaps not very clear. The patient will therefore have reached some sort of conclusion already. In all this there will probably also be a great deal of fear, anger, guilt and any number of other possible emotions.

   A straight, simple question is therefore like a digest of all these factors. To give a simple answer to it may be like putting a match to a heap of timber and causing an explosion.

2. *What is the meaning of it?* The patient will probably not be as concerned with his actual death as what this suffering, illness, physical and emotional pain is all about. Someone concerned with finding meaning or significance is not concerned with details.

   It is therefore better to help the patient to voice his fears and pains, and thus see the meaning. The 'problem' – if he is dying – then somehow solves itself.

3. *What is your goal?* Why did the patient ask the question? Probably not because of any concern at this moment about the minutiae of dying, but to make sense of what is ahead.

   The concern should therefore probably be to help such people come to their own conclusions and in their own time.

4. *How are you going to do it?* When patients have the emotional wherewithal to cope with dying, then, like Mrs Todd, they can begin to think of the practicalities of dying and take the necessary steps to get the information in the ways most appropriate to them (Jones, 1989).

'Never telling a lie' does not mean that you should always tell 'the truth'. What is truth to you may not be the same to the patient, whose truth comes out of experience of living with disease and illness. Your truth may come out of the case-notes and pathology reports; the truths are not necessarily the same. This shows most clearly why it is so important to respond to the *person*, not the problem.

Bereavement   Grieving after death is only different in context from grieving before death. Both aspects mourn something lost. The dying person mourns a personal loss of life, health and all that is important then. The bereaved person mourns the loss of the beloved one's life. The stages of both processes are remarkably similar.

An illness often brings back a multitude of memories (see p. 22), and losses are the strongest memories. Many people are grieving for people and things lost ten, twenty, fifty years earlier. It may not be evident at once that that is the problem, but as soon as you touch on the meaning of a present crisis, the possibility of unfinished grief is very real.

I should like to draw your attention to two aspects here. Women who have had either a stillbirth or an abortion may never have been able, allowed, or allowed themselves, to grieve.

The traumas surrounding stillbirths and perinatal deaths have been recognized more readily recently. Self-help groups and advice centres exist for women and families in this type of bereavement. But still the effects may last for many years and be devastating.

Women who have had abortions may never receive any kind of help. The decision to have an abortion is often a quick one, taken when the person is under pressure. An abortion can literally be done in the lunch-break and nobody need know about it. It may only be years later that the effects are felt, when the person may be feeling too shy, guilty, or helpless to talk about it. A non-judgemental attitude could then be the key to unloading a great deal of grief and freeing the person to live more satisfyingly again.

Spiritual aspects

Coming face to face with one's own mortality may raise questions about spiritual and religious matters. For many patients, and nurses, this is not something with which they are familiar.

When you are listening to a person, you will be hearing what a person is about. You may be able to point to something spiritual which the person might not have recognized. Or the patient may talk to you about God, and that is not an easy subject for you. The genuineness, warmth and empathy required for all counselling are most needed here too, where often one's bias and own needs are most obvious (Kirkpatrick, 1988).

When counselling has failed

Sometimes patients will erect a great variety of defences against help. They go along with you, to please you, but then comes a point when they can take no more. They may say, 'I don't know why I am telling you all this. It's not a problem really'. Or when talking about their families, they suddenly switch and ask, 'Do you have a family?' in order to avoid recalling and dealing with what is perhaps a painful family memory. Or patients may go all the way to seeing a way forward and setting goals, but then simply fail to carry them out. This differs from the reluctance described in Chapter 11; a more unconscious element is at work here, rather like a powerful stopper.

Carkhuff (1969) pointed out that counselling is always 'for better or for worse'; it is never neutral. Egan (1986) is quite sure that it is not the helping *process* which is at fault, but the helpers.

When counselling has not been successful, when the patient gets worse rather than better or refuses to speak to you any more, then it is easy to take all the blame yourself. This is another reason for supervision. It is very important to be as aware as possible when helping, so as to be able to distinguish between what is your problem and what is the client's. No situation is totally black or white, but a great many factors (Moorey and Greer, 1989) are involved in counselling, including the personalities involved, the environment, the health or illness present, the way any referral was handled, etc.

Failure has sometimes to be accepted, and it is painful for both parties. The difficulty is only when it is allowed to become a blockage to further growth.

Referral

One of the things most people need to learn early on is that they have limits. As a nurse and a counsellor you can help some, but not others. You can do so much, but not everything. You will sooner or later come across situations which are beyond your skills. But at least you have uncovered the problem.

Any referral should only be made in the patient's best interest. Those patients who have trusted you with parts of themselves and their lives may find it difficult to confide in someone else. You should therefore be quite sure why a referral is made, or suggested. It may be that you realize that the problem presented is clearly the province of somebody else, such as a social worker, chaplain or psychiatrist. Unless there is good reason not to, you should seek specialist help where applicable.

When referral is the appropriate way forward in a counselling situation, this should be discussed with the client, whose consent to it is necessary. But even when someone else may do most of the counselling, you should still be around, if possible, with care and concern, and not cut the client off completely. A referral may not be available straight away, and so you may need to help the patient not only to accept other help, but to make the transition, and to cover the period between the two helpers.

Nurse (1980) suggests that we should help the clients to make their own application for referral. When you can lead people, through counselling, to manage their own problem, including where to go for specialist help, then the helping process has come full circle. One final aspect of referral is that it

must not be seen as failure on the counsellor's part. On the contrary, it is an ingredient of the whole process of helping, and skill is needed to identify when this is the most appropriate step to take. (Nurse, 1980)

If you have discovered the problem in the first place, then you have done the most important part of the work.

Difficult situations are only one aspect of work; they are only that part of it which give you cause for concern. The other aspects are all the situations which give you joy, and job satisfaction, and make you feel good. But as always, for wholeness in life, both are needed, both challenge us to greater things.

14 Ethical issues

Some basic concepts of ethics

Ethics is not only the study of right and wrong. It also asks *why* right and wrong, and right and wrong in relation to what?

The *Oxford English Dictionary* describes ethics as 'the science of morals; study of the principles of human duty'. Frequently, morals and ethics are equated, yet there are important differences between the two.

> Morality is generally defined as behaviour according to customs or tradition. Ethics, by contrast, is the free, rational assessment of courses of action in relation to principles, rules and conduct. (Churchill, 1977)

Sigman (1979) states that morality is based on culture, and that the culture influences the teaching of morals, and that therefore 'moral development is sequential, observable, and eventual'. But

> to be ethical a person must take the additional step of exercising critical, rational judgement in his decision. He must ask, 'is my customary behaviour right, or good?' (Churchill, 1977)

'Morals' has come to be used in English as one's personal behaviour, and 'ethics' refers to the relationships between human beings. Counselling is therefore deeply associated with ethics, as counselling often challenges these relationships. The helping professions, according to Campbell (1984),

> profess to deal with people not simply by the rules of fair trading (as any seller of services should), but also by an ethic of 'respect for persons'.

This constitutes the right and the wrong in the ethics of counselling, right and wrong in relation to people.

There are two broad strands in ethics. The first is *deontology* (the science of duty or 'ought'), also referred to as non-consequentialism, and known as formalism in the USA; it focuses on rights, duties and principles. This is the philosophical branch of ethics, which is also concerned with establishing codes of ethics. The other strand is *teleology* (the science of final causes), also known as consequentialism or utilitarianism. This area focuses on the actions which produce the greatest good. Much of medical ethics, and indeed the establishment of the National Health Service, rests on this theory.

Despite differences, both orientations are accepted by philosophers as worthy of serious consideration. Both strive to be logical and consistent, and to yield similar decisions in morally similar situations (Candee and Puka, 1984).

A way of combining these two large areas, and seeing not their differences but their complementarity, is to divide the study of ethics into principles. These 'general' principles can then be applied to particular areas, such as medicine, education, business or (as here) counselling. Thiroux (1980) established five such principles: the principle of the value of life; the principle of goodness or rightness; the principle of justice and fairness; the principle of truth telling or honesty and the principle of individual freedom. These overlap and interact. Together they cover the theory of moral behaviour, and they are applicable both to individuals and in general, as will be shown here.

The principle of the value of life

Thiroux sums up this principle with the simple phrase: 'Human beings should revere life and accept death'. Most of the world's moral systems have some prohibition on killing. Those people who value (human) life as a good in itself will want to be sure that they are not killed, and they will not kill others. This principle is, however, infringed in certain situations. Generally speaking these are: abortion, euthanasia, killing in self-defence, war, capital punishment and suicide.

Nurses are mainly concerned with the issues of abortion, euthanasia and suicide. You may not only be caring for patients in these situations but be counselling patients and colleagues who want or have had abortions, who want euthanasia, or who have tried to commit suicide.

Whatever you feel about abortion, euthanasia or suicide will colour the reactions you have when talking with a client about these subjects. Your own personal, philosophical and religious standards matter, and to maintain your integrity you need to be true to these principles. In helping another individual you are not imposing your views but empowering them to find their own personal, philosophical and religious standards. Empathy is going down into the ditch (see Chapter 9), but not taking over. It has also been said that

it is not putting yourself into another's shoes that is morally relevant, (but) it is understanding what it is like for that other person to be in his or her own shoes that is morally important. (Gillon, 1986)

The principle of goodness or rightness

Whichever system of ethics you use, if you want to act ethically, you should strive to be a 'good' human being and attempt to perform 'right' actions. This is easier said than done. What or who is a good person, and in relation to what is that person good? And who establishes good, and who judges it? In all these principles, and here in particular, the question is, to what or to whom do we refer our system of ethics and morality? Who or what is the Absolute against which we measure ourselves and our actions? For some this is God, for others a Supreme Law. It is always something higher than ourselves.

In order to live in a harmonious world, Thiroux (1980) maintains,

human beings attempt to do three things: 1, promote goodness over badness; 2, cause no harm or badness; and 3, prevent badness or harm.

In nursing and counselling this is based on the various professional Codes. The *Code of Professional Conduct for the Nurse, Midwife and Health Visitor* (United Kingdom Central Council, 1984) and the *Code of Ethics and Practice for Counsellors* (British Association for Counselling, 1984) are two such documents. By dealing with issues of responsibility, integrity, competence and confidentiality, both personally and professionally, such codes lay down parameters within which the person should function so that both the individual professional and the profession, the individual client and society at large, benefit, and good is actively promoted and bad or harm prevented.

The principle of justice and fairness

The moral assumptions underlying medical ethics are rarely in dispute. It is in the application of these assumptions to specific cases that the disputes arise. (Campbell and Higgs, 1982)

The principle of socialism, 'from each according to his abilities, to each according to his needs' (Marx), seems indeed just and fair. The difficulty is that 'all animals are equal but some animals are more equal than others' (Orwell). The benefits of being good and doing right should be distributed among people equally and fairly. Thiroux believes that there are three ways in which this can be done:

1, distributing good and bad among people on the basis of their merits; 2, distributing good and bad among people equally; and 3, distributing good and bad to people according to their needs or abilities or both.

The second option is the most egalitarian. The textbook examples of this principle generally concern medicine: if there are only so many kidney machines, or heart transplants, or in vitro fertilizations available, but many more patients need them or deserve them, who should get them? The suggestion is that an impartially conducted lottery would be the most just and fair way to distribute the benefits of good and right.

This is rather utopian. But how do you maintain justice when you are trying to help a person in a dilemma which may involve 'taking from Paul to give to Peter'? Justice is a relative term, and Aristotle argued that 'equals should be treated equally and unequals unequally in proportion to the relevant inequalities' (Gillon, 1986), meaning that those who need more (help) should get it, without thereby taking away anything from anybody.

The principle of truth telling or honesty

Our whole moral system rests on telling the truth. Unless we are sure to be given truthful information, life itself would be untenable. Even when we buy a packet of tea we need to be sure that there is tea in it, and not something else. Equally, you need to pay with honest (real) money, not counterfeit.

In medicine, 'the patient has a *legal right* (author's italics) to expect his medical adviser to take all proper steps to elucidate the truth about his condition' (Duncan et al, 1981). This is the doctor's duty. The difficulty arises when truth telling is not a legal right but an ethical duty.

This principle is infringed by any untruth, white lie, insincerity or misrepresentation. The age-old question, 'What is truth?' would not still be a question if there were a simple answer to it. Henderson (1935) put it wisely;

You can do harm by the process that is quaintly called telling the truth. You can do harm by lying. It will also arise from what you say and from what you fail to say. But try to do as little harm as possible.

The principle of individual freedom

Morality cannot exist if human beings are not to some extent free to make moral choices and decisions. The principles of ethics are therefore only *near* absolutes. Human beings are unique and individual, and therefore have the opportunity to express themselves individually, in and through their lives, and particularly in relationships with other individual human beings. They would have neither individuality nor freedom if the ethical principles were absolutes. But neither freedom itself, nor even moral freedom, is absolute.

As free individuals, we are also autonomous. But autonomy does not mean unconditional freedom. Benjamin and Curtis (1981) say that

Ethical autonomy involves thinking *for* oneself, not *of* oneself or *by* oneself. Thinking *for* oneself is usually more successful if it includes at least some thinking *with* others. One may perfectly well think *for* oneself and still think *about* and *with* others.

This principle stresses equality: the equality of people in moral matters. The Golden Rule, 'do unto others as you would be done by', stresses this point of equality in moral matters. Despite the fact that we are not all social, religious or economic equals, we are all morally equal as persons. The first four principles, of the value of life, goodness, justice and honesty, give us a moral framework, and within them we need to be free to express our individuality, our freedom, and our equality.

This principle is particularly relevant in helping and counselling. As a helper you have the freedom to give or withhold help, when and to whom you give it. Your choice should therefore be a moral one.

You are in a position of influence. The client, by the very fact of being a client, is vulnerable. How you use your influence is therefore crucial.

Without thinking about it and without perhaps realizing it, you are constantly making ethical decisions. This should not be a cause for alarm but, in the spirit of 'the portrait of a helper' (see p. 2), should lead you to constantly greater awareness and the general commitment to your own personal and professional growth. As you review your techniques of helping, so you review your values, and your ethical principles in and of helping.

Personal values and convictions

By caring you respond to something that matters. Your caring matters, and the 'other' that you respond to matters. The way in which you react expresses your feelings. An affective response to someone or something is not emotivism. 'It is an intentional response, deliberate, meaningful and rational' (Roach, 1987).

That response stems out of a person's conscience. 'Conscience grows out of experience, out of a process of valuing self and others. Conscience is the call of care and manifests itself as care' (Roach, 1987). Conscience is more than 'the censorship of morals' (Gillon, 1986); it is the basis and the direction of that which we live by: our values and convictions.

When people have reached a 'moment of truth' which may bring them to ask for help, this is likely to be a moment when their values are suddenly questioned or overturned. What counted until now simply does not count any more. A process of discovery of new values, new meanings and new goals has to start. That is often not possible on one's own.

As a helper you are not in such a crisis. Your own values and way of being may therefore act as a guideline to help other individuals find their own way. However, somewhere, some time in the past you will also have had your 'moment of truth', when you were tested, buffeted and had to grope for new light. This may be the basis for that certain humility that helpers need, in order to 'identify' with their clients. It may also be your strength, because you have come through it and can use that fact as an encouragement to your client, by sharing (see p. 88) some of your experience.

The value of any experience lies in its meaning. The values and convictions you hold are the expressions of the meanings in your life. When these are used in the service of others then you are not only a 'potent' counsellor; you are also an ethical helper.

Standards of care

As the language and concepts of the market place are creeping ever more into health care, nurses may have to ask themselves more clearly where their values lie. Economy, efficiency and effectiveness are definitions of value for money which the Audit Commission is now applying to many areas of the National Health Service (Hodges, 1990).

Every nurse is concerned about the standards of care given. It is difficult to define exactly what a standard is, therefore much depends on the individual nurse and on her concepts and values of caring. The personal integrity of each nurse is therefore vitally important.

The common foundation programmes of Project 2000 courses feature such subjects as respect and dignity, and partnership in caring. If these are taught as subjects from the beginning, then there may be clashes of ideology somewhere when the nurses go to the communities and wards and there find the driving force to be value for money.

It is not easy to maintain concepts of respect for the person in the light of Stock Exchange statistics. Showing respect through attention, confidentiality, advocacy, collaborative relationships and conflict management are rarely measurable in pounds and pence. On the contrary, dealing with these issues takes much nursing time. Yet 'nurturing, comforting, caring, encouraging and facilitating' is what makes nursing 'unique' (Pearson, 1983) and recognizable among other jobs and professions. It is this emotional style (see p. 21) which patients look for and need. On the other hand, measuring nursing care simply in the number of tears shed (Charnock, 1985) is neither possible nor moral. But sometimes, little care and few words but 'being with' is more precious and helpful than any amount of gadgetry.

The profession demands of its workers that they maintain certain levels or standards of care. How they are maintained is the personal duty of each professional. In the area of helping and counselling this may sometimes have to be done by challenging concepts and ideals.

When you believe that human values are as important
as those of the money market, then you may sometimes
have to say so very clearly. But the language of the
marketeer is very different from that of the pastor. To
make yourself heard you may have to learn some of that
other language, while not compromising yours. The only
thing that is sure is that when the moment of truth comes
for a marketeer, he will want to be treated in a person-
centred way, not in a value-for-money way!

Nurses as   The nurse as patient advocate is an idea which is receiving
advocates   a fair amount of interest nowadays. There are obvious
differences between an advocate and a counsellor, but as
a nurse you are likely to be either one, or both, at
different times. It therefore seems reasonable to pay some
attention to this issue. Curtin (1979) bases the concept of
advocacy in

the basic nature and purpose of the nurse–patient
relationship, which in turn is based upon our common
humanity, our common needs and our common human
rights. We are human beings, our patients or clients
are human beings, and it is this commonality that
should form the basis of the relationship between us.

A dictionary definition of an advocate may be one who
pleads for another. The nurse as advocate pleads the
cause of the patient. Unfortunately, this has largely come
to mean fighting the 'system' (Kosik, 1972). In the above
terms advocacy is more subtle.

According to Brown (1985), there are four broad areas
where patient advocacy is called for; these correspond to
the principles of ethics outlined above: (1) in the quality
of care which the patient receives (the principles of the
value of life, and of goodness and right); (2) in the right
and access to care which each patient should have (the
principle of justice and fairness); (3) in full information
which he should receive (the principle of truth telling
and honesty); and (4) in the area of alternatives to care
(the principle of individual freedom). Brown suspects
that 'too often, the only alternative offered to treatment
is no treatment. The patient is thus faced with making
an impossible decision'.

When patients have received full information, then
they may not need someone who pleads their cause, but
someone who gives them the opportunity to discover,

explore and clarify the alternatives so that through them they can live 'more resourcefully and satisfyingly'.

The reverse may be true, too: a nurse discovers, through counselling, that a patient is not receiving quality of care, or the full information, or is not involved enough in the process of care, and the nurse then becomes the patient's advocate. In that sense advocacy may become 'fighting the system'.

Walsh (1985) points out that nurses who act as advocates have the problem of a split in loyalties.

> When a nurse takes on the role of advocate she must consider not only the patient, but her own career, her relationship with the doctor, and the need of her employer. Being an advocate is not a neutral role.

Walsh goes on to say that many nurses would see it as the ultimate objective to lead patients to 'self-advocacy', possibly through pressure groups. Self-advocacy thus coincides with the concept of self-responsibility and having the necessary self-help skills, with the client setting his own goals and striving towards them.

These are not easy issues to tackle. The essence of all interacting between nurses and patients must ultimately rest on the relationship and on human rights, *not* human wants, but real, fundamental human needs (Curtin, 1979).

Nurses as change agents

Whenever you influence something, you change it. Egan (1986) suggests that counselling is a 'social-influence process' and that helpers do this by their attractiveness, trustworthiness and competence. By attractiveness he means a 'perceived similarity to, compatibility with, and liking for the helper'. By trustworthiness he means 'a reputation for honesty, social role (such as doctor, or nurse), sincerity and openness, and lack of motivation for personal gain'. By competence he means 'objective evidence (such as diplomas), behavioural evidence (such as knowledge and confidence), and reputation as an expert'.

In one Project 2000 programme one of the human skills areas to be learnt is 'partnership in caring' and that involves demonstrating effective communication skill, acting as advocate for the patient or client, managing conflict constructively, and showing assertiveness in action. These are essentially the skills of effective change agents: people who do not accept the status quo simply

because someone said so, or because they are too timid;
people who so passionately care for others that they will
speak up for them; people who strive for a better
environment wherever this is possible by uncovering
conflict and facing it constructively.

These are not only nursing skills. They are also
basic communication skills. Above all they are helping
(counselling) skills.

Accountability

Accountability is often linked with economy and saving
money. You are accountable for the number of syringes
you use and the number of hours you spend 'talking'.

To be accountable, you must have authority to act.

This can be an authority based on conscience and
ethical values (moral accountability) and that based on
professional competence (legal accountability). In either
case there must be a basis in knowledge which can be
explained and defended. (Tschudin, 1989a)

It is evident that legal, or economic, accountability sits
uneasily with counselling. But moral accountability is
something which all counsellors know. In this type of
accountability the line goes not to the next higher manager
(and so on to the top), but the accountability is always
to the client, in whatever setting. This is not a case of
'the client is always right'; it is a case of this accountability
stemming from a respect for the person, and the needs
of that person.

In practice this may mean that the working or caring
relationship you have with a person is of paramount
importance and that nobody has any right to change this,
or interfere with it. If this is so, the need for good
professional supervision becomes even more evident.

**Confidentiality
and
documentation**

As one aspect of helping leads to another and depends
on another, so it can be seen that confidentiality is
necessarily the next step from moral accountability. When
you respect both the person of the client and the
relationship which you have, then confidentiality is that
which keeps the trust.

Unless patients know they can trust their nurse, they
are unlikely to talk about themselves. Sometimes you
may need to give patients the assurance beforehand that
anything said between you is indeed between you only.

If possible, you should then ensure that no one else overhears, something not so easily achieved in, for example, a hospital ward.

Confidentiality has wide implications. Not only do wards have ears; hospital dining rooms and buses have all been the scenes of unwitting disclosures by nurses, sometimes with disastrous consequences. If you talk about your work, you should be quite sure that you do not do it in such a manner that the patient is recognized, anyhow, anywhere.

A patient may not consider what was said to be confidential. Indeed, in many instances it is not particularly confidential, but that should never be an excuse for gossip.

Occasionally you may hear disturbing facts related by patients. There may be some very good reasons why individuals chose to reveal a certain aspect of themselves, or a deed they have done. You have to be not only unshockable, but sometimes have to live with disturbing knowledge.

Occasionally it is not possible, for one reason or another, to keep something confidential. It is then not only courteous but essential that the patient knows what you are going to do, and that such an action is consented to.

It is becoming more and more usual for patients to see their casenotes or to take part in hand-over reports. What is said and written has, therefore, not only to be accurate, but actually helpful to the patient. This makes confidentiality an even more important aspect of care. What you say and how you say it can make the difference between help and hindrance.

To say (or write) that you had a talk with a patient is often helpful because it may make your relationship legitimate in the eyes of your colleagues. It may also help the other members of staff to respect your relationship with that particular patient. And knowing that you are the patient's 'counsellor' may indeed relieve other colleagues from a sense of duty, by knowing that one of their number has taken that aspect seriously.

Counselling and the institution

Most nurses who have and use counselling skills work in institutions or agencies of one kind or another. And, since counselling is a social-influence process, by sheer dint of *doing* counselling they influence people and systems around them. Yet many nurses find that their organization is 'alienating', i.e., it is a 'social order which is "remote", incomprehensible or fraudulent; beyond hope or desire; inviting apathy, boredom or even hostility' (Nisbet, 1969). It is hardly surprising that many nurses see their organization as something that is against them; therefore they can only be against it in return. Yet because they work in it, they also need it and use it.

Jameton (1984) talks of moral problems in nursing, and reserves the strongest type, moral distress, for situations 'when one knows the right thing to do, but institutional constraints make it nearly impossible to pursue the right course of action'.

When using counselling skills openly with patients and colleagues you may come in conflict with the organization. You are told you spend too much time 'just talking'; you upset colleagues by your loyalties; and you may find that if you would like to create a more adequate atmosphere of support, you are heading for trouble with the institution as such.

Equally, the institution, the senior personnel, may feel that you are doing something which is not strictly in your job description, and for which permission has not been given. Either way, there is conflict, and eventually distress. This may be made more acute by the mere fact that you are actually trying to help someone.

On the other hand, counselling and helping are being seen more and more as important elements in nursing. Yet, alone, you cannot change the institution to subscribe to this form of care; but you can influence the institution.

When you believe that using counselling and helping skills in health care settings is better than not using them, not only will individual patients benefit, but the system itself will become less alienated, less remote, more comprehensible, more 'healthy' and more contented. As you cannot do this single-handedly, you need to do it in a way which the organization understands.

Egan and Cowan (1979) believe 'systems influence systems, and people may influence systems best through other systems'. You need to understand how systems work, and what your sphere of influence is. A charge nurse who uses counselling and helping skills consciously will be creating an atmosphere of trust in the ward. Gradually, more nurses will want to work there.

As a nurse you can influence the system by promoting counselling, seeking the skills, acquiring them and using them. In the Project 2000 training, these skills are deemed essential, but it will be some time before nurses have been trained and can use their skills in this way throughout the health care system, time in which help *can* be given and suffering relieved by being truly 'with' patients and clients – being companions on the road with them.

Ethical issues are not something extra or different from helping and caring in general. The caring nurse is inevitably an ethical nurse, and vice versa. What may be new is the language of some of the concepts. What remains is that at the centre there is a person with needs – and that could be you one day, which may be a sobering thought in terms of duty, or responsibility, and your response to suffering in general.

15 Nurses counselling nurses

The nurse as counsellor

Nurses who learn about counselling often ask what the specific skills are in counselling people with cancer, or AIDS, or who are dying, or children, or other 'special' groups. I believe that there is essentially no difference in the counselling skills used for any person or speciality. The skills are the same; the process is the same. The only thing which is different is the context, and perhaps the language used, particularly for children.

Some individuals have an affinity for certain groups of people, and this should be exploited where possible. Nurses who specialize in a particular field do so because it suits their character and temperament, and therefore they are naturally (or potentially) good in that field. This does not necessarily apply to colleagues. There is a completely different relationship with colleagues, which gives the whole area of helping colleagues a different ethos.

Tutor-counsellors

Nurses who adopt a combined tutor-counsellor role may find themselves faced with multiple moral dilemmas arising from their contact with learners. Can they keep faith with their responsibility of providing information to the nursing school or administration, and yet keep a total counselling commitment of confidence to nurse learners? (Bailey, 1981)

As soon as there is any counselling done by people who are in a hierarchical relationship to each other, the dynamics of counselling change. Issues such as confidentiality, documentation and referral become immediately obvious.

On entry into nursing a young person is allocated to a tutor who has that student's welfare particularly in mind. There may be other such 'special' people for the new student, such as a mentor or a more senior nurse. These people are then not only their teachers, but take on a mother role. For some students, especially very young people, this may be ideal, but for others it may be a cause for confusion. When a problem arises, they feel obliged to go to their tutor who they may respect as a teacher but would not like to pour their heart out to. Where else are they to go?

A sensitive tutor is aware of these possible pitfalls, and in many schools of nursing and campuses systems are in operation where a student chooses the tutor he or she most easily relates to.

Nevertheless, the issue remains how far a student can take a personal problem to a tutor without it interfering in her or his academic career. When does a personal problem become a career problem?

The tutor in the dialogue below made it clear, during discussions following lectures on ethics, that she was against abortion. Nevertheless, she found herself again and again in the position of helping students who had become pregnant. The following is an extract from one such interview, which started at 4 p.m. on a Friday:

Student: (knocks) Can I come in?

Tutor: Of course. My, you look dreadful, what's up?

Student: I haven't slept for a week.

Tutor: Before you tell me why, can I say that I have about twenty minutes.

Student: Ten will be enough.

Tutor: Well, let's see. You haven't slept?

Student: To cut a long story short, I got suspicious and had a pregnancy test the other day which confirmed my worst fears. I guess I'm about ten weeks.

Tutor: Go on.

Student: My boyfriend doesn't want to know. He says I'm the nurse, and I ought to have been more careful.

Tutor: He doesn't want to know?

Student: I – I . . . You see . . . The worst part . . . I don't trust him . . . .

Tutor: Mm?

Student: I don't think he is reliable.

Tutor: Reliable?

Student: He's knocked about a bit. He boasts rather about his experiences.

Tutor: Sowing wild oats?

Student: (breaking into tears) More than that, really, HIV . . . I can't help wondering.

Tutor: It sounds as if *that* is the worst bit.

Student: (drying her tears) You guessed.

Tutor: Well, that's quite a story. I don't think we're going to solve it in ten minutes.

Student: (smiles) Thanks. I was desperate. I just had to come.

Tutor: I appreciate that, and I'm glad you did come. Let's see how I can best help you in the time we've left.

Student: Well, you've helped me already by letting me talk. I've made up my mind I want an abortion. I know you don't agree. But I want to continue with nursing. I couldn't face my mother if I didn't. She is dead against abortion too.

Tutor: You sound as if your mind is made up.

Student: I think so.

Tutor: You're not sure?

Student: I never had to face the issue before. I had thought of myself as rather shy and traditional, and even a coward. I hardly know myself and my reactions now.

Tutor: It's never easy to make a big decision which will affect your life at a time when you are under pressure and not sure of your standpoint.

Student: Do you think I should wait?

Tutor: In what way could waiting help you?

Student: It would prolong the agony. But we could also talk things over a bit more.

Tutor: We?

Student: My boyfriend and I.

Tutor: It's sometimes helpful to set a goal, say giving yourself so many days in which to decide.

Student: Oh, that's a good idea. I think next Friday I would need to know.

Tutor: That's good. That gives you time to think of the alternatives. Who else could you talk it over with, to give you another viewpoint?

Student: I can go to M. She's a bit older than I am but she's always been a good friend, and she's not stuffy.

Tutor: Does that feel easier now?

Student: (letting out a long sigh) A lot.

Tutor: Where do you go from now?

Student: I'm going home now to phone my boyfriend. Then I'll call M. Can I come to you again if I need to?

> *Tutor*: Of course, with pleasure.
> *Student*: And I'll let you know in any case what I decide. Thanks a million.

The twenty minutes was just about up. The student did have an abortion. The fact that she had a mother and a tutor who were both against abortion made her face her own values more clearly. She had decided that the meaning of her life was essentially in nursing at the moment. The tutor did not put any pressure on her; by offering her the idea of a deadline, the student could see a way forward and knew how to go that way.

Figure 15.1 shows the conversation in relation to the three models and the four questions outlined. As you read it, you might like to decide for yourself which helper attitudes (e.g. non-judgemental) and skills (e.g. reflection, challenging) are used and where.

Manager-counsellors

Manager-counsellors encounter similar pitfalls to tutor-counsellors, except that they deal with qualified staff, not students.

The great difficulty with manager-counsellors is the ambiguity of the language. Is a manager able to counsel, or is he or she disciplining? The junior member in the hierarchy, when called to see the line manager, may be suspicious.

> They may feel that it is not counselling per se, but a form of appraisal, whereby they are encouraged to change their attitudes and behaviours – to think things out for themselves so long as they come to the conclusions desired by the counsellor. (Salaman, 1983)

Managers are inevitably called upon in cases of discipline. It is easy then to call it 'counselling', as it will sound less severe. The fact is that neither party is helped by that, because discipline still has to be upheld, and counselling did not happen.

Hore (1984) defines managers as people who must achieve results through others; and counselling as a non-directive process that helps people to help themselves. These two approaches to people essentially complement each other. When, therefore, a manager-counsellor has objectives other than those of the organization or of education, he or she embarks on the slippery slope to manipulation, which is a seductive trap for any manager.

Figure 15.1

EGAN NELSON-JONES | CARKHUFF TSCHUDIN

Problem definition (Present scenario)

[De]scribe and identify the problem

D

Student: (knocks) Can I come in?
Tutor: Of course. My, you look dreadful, what's up?
S: I haven't slept for a week.
T: Before you tell me why, can I say that I have about 20 minutes.
S: Ten will be enough.
T: Well, let's see. You haven't slept?
S: To cut a long story short, I got suspicious and had a pregnancy test the other day which confirmed my worst fears. I guess I'm about ten weeks.
T: Go on.
S: My boyfriend doesn't want to know. He says I'm the nurse, and I ought to have been more careful.
T: He doesn't want to know . . .?
S: I – I . . . You see . . . The worst part . . . I don't trust him either . . . .
T: Mm . . .?
S: I don't think he is reliable.
T: Reliable?
S: He's knocked about a bit. He boasts about his experiences.
T: Sowing wild oats?
S: More than that really (breaking into tears) . . . HIV . . . I can't help wondering.
T: It sounds as if *that* is the worst bit.
S: You guessed (drying her tears).
T: Well, that's quite a story. I don't think we're going to solve it in ten minutes.
S: (smiles) Thanks. I was desperate, I just had to come.
T: I appreciate that, and I'm glad you did come. Let's see how I can best help you in the time we've left.
S: Well, you've helped me already by letting me talk. I've made up my mind I want an abortion. I know you don't agree. But I

Attending

Responding to client

What is happening?

I didn't. She is dead against abortion too. I couldn't face my mother if

T: You sound as if your mind is made up.

S: I think so.

T: You're not sure?

S: I never had to face the issue before. I had thought of myself as rather shy and traditional, and even a coward. I hardly know myself and my reactions now.

T: It's never easy to make a big decision which will affect your life at a time when you are under pressure and not sure of your standpoint.

S: Do you think I should wait?

T: In what way would waiting help you?

S: It would prolong the agony. But we could also talk things over a bit more.

T: We?

S: My boyfriend and I.

T: It's sometimes helpful to set a goal, say giving yourself so many days in which to decide.

S: Oh, that's a good idea. I think I would need to know by next Friday.

T: That's good. That gives you time to think of the alternatives. Who else could you talk it over with, to give you another point of view?

S: I can go to M. She's a bit older than I am but she's always been a good friend and she's not stuffy.

T: Does that feel easier now?

S: (letting out a long sigh) A lot.

T: Where do you go from now?

S: I'm going home now to phone my boyfriend. Then I'll call M. Can I come to you again, if I need to?

T: Of course, with pleasure.

S: And I'll let you know in any case what I decide. Thanks a million.

Exit and consolidate self-help skills

Operationalize the problem

Set goals

Intervene

Goal development (Future scenario)

Action

When a manager can make it clear to the client which of the two approaches is being used, then clarity will be not only maintained, but fostered, and both sides will benefit.

Yet it is not possible for a manager in an interview to say 'Now I am managing' (i.e. concerned with the organization) or 'Now I am counselling' (i.e. helping the client to help himself). A good manager, like a good helper, will concentrate on the individual, not on the problem.

The aim is not to solve one particular problem but to assist the individual to *grow*, so that he can cope with the present problem and with later problems in a better integrated fashion. (Rogers, 1978)

More and more organizations realize that their personnel function best when encouraged to take part in decisions and when these decisions are then tried and implemented. When 'power to the people' is not only a slogan but a working maxim, then a manager-counsellor will be using counselling skills to help the workforce to help themselves; and managerial skills to get the best for the organization. Then he or she is using power most helpfully.

Colleague-counsellors

Unfortunately, it is all too often true that 'nurses seem to regard any sign of stress in an individual as unacceptable and if ignored it may go away' (Moore, 1984). Much of this is due to the nursing culture. There is a tradition in nursing which seems to think that unless we punish, discipline and correct, 'they' will not become 'good nurses'.

The Briggs Report (Committee on Nursing, 1972) found that 'many ward sisters, tutors and nursing officers provide support as do hospital chaplains'. But such help is *ad hoc*. This may be precisely why it is chosen. Anything more long-term could easily be regarded as therapy.

Most of the helping done by colleagues happens at points of crises. It is impossible to be alongside pain and suffering all day without being affected by it. Much of the care given is at great personal cost – rightly; and sometimes wrongly. 'You see them when the patient keeps ringing the bell and they grimace to themselves. Then they go up to the patient all smiles' (Smith, 1989).

At some stage, a breaking point is reached and the lid comes off. The first to catch what is coming out is a colleague. Helping each other in such situations is not only necessary, but often very beneficial for relationships all round.

But can it be done long-term? And officially? Counselling colleagues can lead into conflicts of loyalties. Is a nurse firstly loyal to 'the hospital (which employs her), the physician (with whom she works), the client (for whom she provides care), or the nursing profession (to which she belongs)?' (Benjamin and Curtis, 1981). Loyalty to colleagues has always been highly prized, which is perhaps why much helping has gone on among colleagues, and not much independent help has either been sought or used. When you are helping colleagues you may have to consider their and your ethical standpoints. 'Loyalty' has sometimes been blamed for blatant disregard of major issues. Nurses were not given realistic help because colleagues covered up. This is precisely where counselling colleagues can turn into a curse when it was meant to be a blessing. It needs to go on; but it needs to go on with eyes wide open and with as much clarity and empathy as can be mustered.

The increasing incidence of drug and alcohol abuse among nurses has often been highlighted (Booth, 1985). The sheer availability of drugs makes nurses vulnerable to abuse, although Booth claims that 'most of the factors influencing alcohol and drug consumption by nurses are unrelated to the nursing profession'. This is significant, because it shows that nurses still take on a persona when they put on their uniform and almost deny that they have another life; and also that nurses have cared very little for each other as *persons*.

Perhaps the most difficult situation is not when a colleagues comes to you with a problem, but when you notice that the colleague has not been as caring or happy as usual, and you suspect a problem. What approach should you take? The following is a reconstruction of a conversation between two staff nurses.

A: Hi, how are you?
B: Hi, OK, how's you?
A: Fine, thanks. Mm . . . you sounded a bit uncheerful just then.
B: Oh? I'm all right.
A: I'm going to be straight. I'm worried about you. Tell me

if it's none of my business, but you *have* been a bit on edge recently.

B: Are you in one of your helpful moods? Because if so, I don't want it.

A: Yes, I guess I am. But we have to work together, and I can't work happily when you go around looking like sour grapes.

B: You can talk, you've got everything you want.

A: You mean, you haven't?

B: All right, you asked for it: I found out my husband has a 'friend' and my mother has got Alzheimer's and I can't cope any more.

A: Well, that's quite a packet.

B: Do you still want to know now?

A: I'm happier to know the reason for your absent-mindedness. What have you done to cope?

B: Nothing.

A: Nothing?

B: It was too much to do anything.

A: Can I help in any way?

B: It's kind of you to offer, but no, thanks.

A: But you are not coping at work either.

B: There are ways and means.

A: And I guess what one of them is, and that is what concerns me most.

B: If you were weren't so b. nice I'd tell you to get lost.

A: I know I'm intruding, but I fear that sooner or later someone will run to the office and tell them but not tell you about it.

B: Yes, I just had to find a solution, and vodka was the easiest one. I don't take a lot though.

A: Enough to make you sleepy and occasionally unsafe at work.

B: (tearful) I tried to hide it.

A: It's not that easy.

B: (crying) I really don't know what to do. My whole life has just collapsed into a heap. I'm not worth anything any more.

A: I can understand you saying that. But I for one respect you as much as ever.

B: Really?

A: Sure, that's why I risked tackling you.

B: (smiles)

A: OK. Where are you going to start?

B: I know what needs doing. I just need to get the courage from somewhere.

A: That's brave of you to think like that.
B: Seeing that you had the courage to tackle me, will you help me to find my courage?
A: With pleasure, as far as I am able to.

Not all such situations are so easy or so successful. The outstanding quality in this helper was her unwavering respect for her colleague, and it was that which was recognized as the empathy which made the connection between helplessness and self-help.

Burnard (1990) writes of the situation of a nurse manager going to a colleague in a more junior position for help and counselling. With more open styles of work, positions get blurred, and with them the traditional boundaries. Yet 'it may be easier for a person in a senior position to talk (more) readily about his problem than it may be for someone junior to adopt the role of counsellor'. Once the culture of the hierarchy has been instilled it is very difficult to remove it again. So the person who is junior may always feel inferior, even though she or he may be many years older than the boss.

When a senior chooses a junior for help there may be many reasons: her age, her experience, her reputation (as a listener), her 'safety' in the sense that she may not have any ambitions to defend, or is known not to talk 'shop'. Whatever the reasons, it is not easy for the helper to be put into this position. But compassion and duty oblige her to stay there, and help in the best way possible. The skills used are the same; the process is the same. What may be different in this situation are the boundaries, what they are, where they are, and what they may mean. Perhaps establishing that may already be half the problem solved.

Counselling colleagues is perhaps one of the most fraught situations a nurse can be in, but also the most challenging.

'We are all in this together' is a cliché; it is also very true. Unless we help each other we don't help our patients. Curtin and Flaherty (1982) say that

one of the most effective ways to promote excellence in nursing practice is for nurses to offer support, guidance, criticism and direction to one another. To fail or to refuse to offer this kind of assistance actually constitutes a breach of faith – not just with colleagues, but also with the public because it will affect negatively the quality of nursing services offered.

And Fromant (1988), writing of the intensive care unit in which she works, says

What has become apparent in our unit is that, as we get to know each other, we develop a sensitivity to the early signals of stress. It is this early warning system and the willingness to respond which is our best defence against stress.

Postscript

A friend said to me recently, 'You're right, hearing is loving'. I looked at him, nonplussed. He was leafing through something I had written, and he showed it to me. There it was, 'Hearing is Loving'. I had forgotten that I had written it. Having it pointed out, and spelled out, made me hear it in a completely new way. It made me ask what I really mean by 'hearing is loving'. My friend said, 'I can listen to someone, but when I hear him then I am with him, and then I love him'.

Loving is not a skill. It can never be a 'technical mastery or a calculated tactic' (Halmos, 1965). Genuine help, says Campbell (1984)

> must see each person, including the helper, afresh, as a new and separate being, for whom no real parallel exists in prior experience – the unique encountering the unique.

Halmos (1965) writes at great length about love in the therapeutic (psychiatric) relationship. He talks of many aspects of loving in that relationship: empathy, rapport, encounter, identity, communion and even the 'I–Thou relationship'. He believes that psychotherapy (he calls the psychotherapists 'counsellors') 'has to be an appropriate mixture of mothering (management) and analysis (giving insight)'. Counselling and helping is not a set of skills; it is knowing what is appropriate, and then doing it.

> . . . years of unsparing friendship between case-worker and client, floral tributes brought along personally to the funeral of client's husband, taking client out to lunches, gifts and presents, and every sign of warm and sustained mutuality . . .. (Halmos, 1965)

Campbell (1984) talks of 'lovers and professors' by saying that certain occupational groups *profess to love*, claiming both the title 'profession' and a commitment to 'service of mankind'. These groups are both 'lovers' and 'professors'. What they profess, in addition to knowledge and skill, *is* a disinterested love. The requirements of disinterested love are that the 'professors' restore 'full value to every individual, however damaged, however oppressed, however bereft of hope'. This may sound like an impossible ideal. Perhaps helping another person will always remain 'impossible' (how can 'help' be measured?), yet also an 'ideal' in the sense that we have to express our humanity in ways which take us forward, and that means that I cannot go forward alone, but only in company with all humanity.

I realize that I personally always look forward, sometimes at the expense of tradition and memory. I could be called an idealist. This necessarily colours how I work, teach and write. Do I love by pulling people forward with me? That would be manipulation. Do I forget the past too much? That would be denial. Counselling *people* challenges me to become more whole myself. Their needs challenge me; I challenge theirs. Thus is love generated and spread around. I cannot help but equate this with 'love your neighbour as yourself', and Halmos (1965) said the same in a few lines which keep ringing in my ears:

'You are worthwhile!' and 'I am not put off by your illness!' This moral stance of not admitting defeat is possible for those who have faith or a kind of stubborn confidence in the rightness of what they are doing. Yet all that the counsellor freely confesses to is a mere technique, an elaborate professional etiquette, or a sheer casuistry of professionalized neighbourliness.

Bibliography

(* Titles recommended for further reading.)

*Aguilera, D. (1986) *Crisis Intervention: Theory and Methodology*. St Louis: C.V. Mosby.

Altschul, A. & Sinclair, H.C. (1981) *Psychology for Nurses*. London: Baillière Tindall.

*Argyle, M. (1981) *Social Skills and Health*. London: Methuen.

Bailey, R. (1981) Counselling services for nurses – a forgotten responsibility. *Apex (Journal of the British Institute of Mental Handicap)* 9(2): 45–47.

Bandler, R. (1985) *Using your Brain – For a Change*. Moab, Utah: Real People Press.

Benjamain, M. & Curtis, J. (1981) *Ethics in Nursing*. New York: Oxford University Press.

Berne, E. (1964) *Games People Play*. Harmondsworth: Penguin.

Blue, L. (1985) *Bright Blue*. London: BBC.

Bond, M. (1979) The use of co-counselling. *Nursing Times* 75(35): 1532 (letter).

Booth, P. (1985) Back on the rails. *Nursing Times* 81(35): 16–17.

*Bowlby, J. (1979) *Making and Breaking of Affectional Bonds*. London: Tavistock.

Bowlby, R.O. (1986) Caring, authority and achievement in large institutions. *Counselling* 56: 8–13.

Brammer, L. (1973) *The Helping Relationship*. Englewood Cliffs, NJ: Prentice Hall.

*Brearley, G. (1986) *Introducing Counselling Skills and Techniques*. London: Faber.

British Association for Counselling (1984) *Code of Ethics*. Rugby: BAC.

British Association for Counselling (1989) *Definition of Counselling*. Rugby: BAC.

Brown, J. (1988) Care of the dying. In Tschudin, V. (ed.) (1988) *Nursing the Patient with Cancer*. Hemel Hempstead: Prentice Hall.

Brown, M. (1985) Matter of commitment. *Nursing Times* **81**(18): 26–27.

*Burnard, P. (1989) *Counselling Skills for Health Professionals*. London: Chapman & Hall.

Burnard, P. (1990) Counselling the boss. *Nursing Times* **86**(1): 58–59.

Burton, G. (1979) *Interpersonal Relations, a Guide for Nurses*. London: Tavistock.

*Campbell, A.V. (1981) *Rediscovering Pastoral Care*. London: Darton, Longman & Todd.

Campbell, A.V. (1984) *Moderated Love*. London: Society for Promoting Christian Knowledge.

Campbell, A.V. & Higgs, R. (1982) *In That Case*. London: Darton, Longman & Todd.

Candee, D. & Puka, B. (1984) An analytic approach to resolving problems in medical ethics. *Journal of Medical Ethics* **10**(2): 61–70.

Carkhuff, R.R. (1969) *Helping and Human Relations*, vol. 1. New York: Holt, Rinehart & Winston.

Carkhuff, R.R. (1987) (6th edn) *The Art of Helping*. Amherst: Human Resource Development Press.

Charles-Edwards, A. (1983) *Nursing Care of the Dying Patient*. Beaconsfield: Beaconsfield Publishers.

Charnock, A. (1985) Sharing the sadness. *Nursing Times* **81**(40): 40–41.

Churchill, L. (1977) Ethical issues of a profession in transition. *American Journal of Nursing* **77**(5): 873–875.

Clark, L. (1978) Counselling, absenteeism and research. *Nursing Times* **74**(31): 1337–1338.

Clarke, L. (1986) Deterioration effects induced by psychological counselling. *Counselling* **57**: 8–13.

*Cleese, J. (1983) *Families and How to Survive Them*. London: Mandarin Octopus.

Committee on Nursing (1972) (Briggs) *Report*. London: HMSO.

Cormack, D. (1985) The myth and reality of interpersonal skills use in nursing. In Kagan, C.M. (ed.) (1985) *Interpersonal Skills in Nursing*. London: Croom Helm.

Cox, C. (1979) Who cares? Nursing and sociology: the development of a symbiotic relationship. *Journal of Advanced Nursing* **4**: 237–252.

Crawley, P. (1983) Call in for a chat. *Nursing Mirror* **156**(14): 510.

Curtin, L. & Flaherty, M.J. (1982) *Nursing Ethics, Theories and Pragmatics.* Bowie, MD: Robert J. Brady.

Curtin, L.L. (1979) The nurse as advocate: a philosophical foundation for nursing. *Advances in Nursing Science* **1**(3): 1–10.

Daniel, J. (1984) 'Sympathy' or 'empathy'? *Journal of Medical Ethics*. **10**(2): 103 (letter).

Davis, K. (1972) In Lancaster, J. & Lancaster, W. (1982) *Concepts for Advanced Nursing Practice*. St Louis: C.V. Mosby.

*Dryden, W. (1984) *Individual Therapy in Britain*. Milton Keynes: Open University Press.

Duncan, A.S., Dunstan, G.R. & Wellbourn, R.B. (1981) *Dictionary of Medical Ethics* (2nd edn). London: Darton, Longman & Todd.

*Egan, G. (1975) *Exercises in Helping Skills*. Belmont, CA: Brooks/Cole.

Egan, G. (1977) *You and Me*. Monterey, CA: Brooks/Cole.

Egan, G. (1982) *The Skilled Helper* (2nd edn). Belmont, CA: Wadsworth Publishing.

Egan, G. (1986) *The Skilled Helper* (3rd edn). Belmont, CA: Wadsworth Publishing.

*Egan, G. (1990) *The Skilled Helper* (4th edn). Belmont, CA: Brooks/Cole.

Egan, G. & Cowan, R.M. (1979) *People and Systems, an Integrative Approach to Human Development*. Belmont, CA: Brooks/Cole.

Eliot, T.S. (1944) *Four Quartets*. London; Faber & Faber.

*Epting, F. (1984) *Personal Construct Counselling and Therapy*. Chichester: Wiley.

Erikson, E.H. (1964) *Childhood and Society* (revised edn). Harmondsworth: Penguin.

Fabun, D. (1968) Communications. In Navone, J. (1977) *Towards a Theology of Story*. Slough: St Paul Publications.

Fast, J. (1971) *Body Language*. London: Pan.

Ferrucci, P. (1982) *What We May Be*. Wellingborough: Thorsons.

Forsyth, G.L. (1979) Exploration of empathy in nurse–client interaction. *Advances in Nursing Science* **1**(2): 53–61.

*Franchino, L. (1989) *Bereavement and Counselling: A Handbook for Trainees*. Weybridge: Counselling Services.

*Franchino, L. (1989) *Bereavement Counsellors Training Manual* (3 volumes). Weybridge: Counselling Services.

Frankl, V. (1962) *Man's Search for Meaning*. London: Hodder & Stoughton.

Fraser, J. (1990) Reading between the lines. *Nursing Times* **86**(5): 45–47.

Fromant, P. (1988) Helping each other. *Nursing Times* **84**(36): 30, 32.

Galbraith, V. (1979) In Egan, G. (ed.) (1986) *The Skilled Helper* (3rd edn). Belmont, CA: Wadsworth Publishing.

Gawain, S. (1978) *Creative Visualization*. New York: Bantam.

*Gersie, A. (1990) *Storymaking in Bereavement*. London: Jessica Kingsley Publishers.

Gilbert, P. (1989) *Human Nature and Suffering*. Hove: Lawrence Erlbaum.

Gillon, R. (1986) *Philosophical Medical Ethics*. Chichester: Wiley.

*Gilmore, S. (1973) *The Counsellor-in-Training*. Englewood Cliffs, NJ: Prentice Hall.

Gilmore, S. (1984) Training in counselling skills. Workshop.

Glasser, W. (1965) *Reality Therapy*. New York: Harper & Row.

Goldman, E.E. & Morrison, D.S. (1984) *Psychodrama: Experience and Process*. Dubuque, IA: Kendall/Hunt.

Halmos, P. (1965) *The Faith of the Counsellors*. London: Constable.

Hancock, C. (1983) The need for support. *Nursing Times* **79**(38): 43–45.

Hargie, O., Saunders, C. & Dickson, D. (1981) *Social Skills in Interpersonal Communications*. London: Croom Helm.

Harris, T.A. (1973) *I'm OK – You're OK*. London: Pan.

Henderson, H.J. (1935) In Duncan, A.S., Dunstan, G.R. & Welbourn, R.B. (eds) (1981) *Dictionary of Medical Ethics*. London: Dalton, Longman & Todd.

Henderson, V. (1966) *The Nature of Nursing*. New York: Macmillan.

Heywood Jones, I. (1989) Buried under paper. *Nursing Times*, **85**(34): 57–58.

Hodges, C. (1990) Value for money. *Nursing Times*, **86**(14): 20.

Hogan, R. (1969) Development of an empathy scale. *Journal of Consulting and Clinical Psychology* **33**(3): 307–316.

Hore, I.D. (1984) Can managers counsel? *Counselling* **48**: 7–13.

*Hughes, J. (1987) *Cancer and Emotion*. Chichester: Wiley.

Inskipp, F. (1985) *A Manual for Trainers*. London: Alexia Publications.

Inskipp, F. & Johns, H. (1984) *Principles of Counselling: Insight*. London: BBC.

*Ivey, A. et al. (1987) *Counselling and Psychotherapy*. Englewood Cliffs, NJ: Prentice Hall.

Jacobs, M. (1982) *Still Small Voice*. London: Society for Promoting Christian Knowledge.

Jameton, A. (1984) *Nursing Practice: the Ethical Issues*. Englewood Cliffs, NJ: Prentice-Hall.

Jesson, A. & Wilmot, V. (1990) Report from the Forum for Nurses working as counsellors. *Newsletters of Counselling in Medical Settings*, No. 22: 8–12.

Jones, C. (1989) Little white lies. *Nursing Times*, **85**(44): 38–39.

Jones, D. (1978) The need for a comprehensive counselling service for nursing students. *Journal of Advanced Nursing* **3**, 359–368.

*Jourard, S.M. (1971) *The Transparent Self*. New York: Van Nostrand Reinhold.

Jung, C.G. (1933) *Modern Man in Search of a Soul*. London: Routledge & Kegan Paul.

Jung, C.G. (1964) *Man and his Symbols*. London: Pan.

Kalisch, B.J. (1971) Strategies for developing nurse empathy. *Nursing Outlook* **19**(11): 714–717.

*Kennedy, E. (1977) *On Becoming a Counsellor*. Dublin: Gill & Macmillan.

*Kennedy, E. (1981) *Crisis Counselling*. Dublin: Gill & Macmillan.

*Kfir, N. (1989) *Crisis Intervention Verbatim*. New York: Hemisphere.

King, J. (1984) A question of attitude. *Nursing Times* **80**(45): 51–52.

Kirkpatrick, B. (1988) *AIDS. Sharing the Pain*. London: Dalton, Longman & Todd.

Kirkpatrick, W. (1985) *Reaching Out*. Private circulation.

Knight, A. (1979) The need for a nurse counsellor at the Royal Marsden Hospital. Study presented for Joint Board of Clinical Nursing Studies Course.

Kosik, S. (1972) in Brown, M. (1985) Matter of commitment. *Nursing Times* **81**(18): 26–27.

Krumboltz, J.D. & Thorenson, C.E. (1969) *Behavioral*

counselling: cases and techniques. New York: Holt, Rinehart & Winston.

Kübler-Ross, E. (1970) *On Death and Dying.* London: Tavistock.

LaMonica, E.L. et al. (1976) Empathy training as the major thrust of a staff development program. *Nursing Research* **25** (6): 447–451.

Lefébure, M. (1985) *Conversations on Counselling.* Edinburgh: T. T. Clarke.

Lefébure, M. (1985) *Human experience and the Art of Counselling.* Edinburgh: T. & T. Clark.

*MacLean, D. (1988) *The Helping Process: An Introduction.* London: Croom Helm.

*Marris, P. (1986) *Loss and Change.* London: Routledge.

Marson, S.N. (1979) Nursing, a helping relationship? *Nursing Times* **75**(13): 541–544.

Martin, I.C.A. (1977) A strident silence. *Nursing Times* **73**(19): 754–755.

Mathews, B.P. (1962) Measurement of psychological aspects of the nurse–patient relationship. *Nursing Research* **11**(3): 154–162.

Mayeroff, M. (1972) *On Caring.* New York: Harper & Row.

Menzies, I. (1960) A case-study in the functioning of social systems as a defence against anxiety. *Human Relations* **13**(2): 95–121.

Miller, W.A. (1981) *Make Friends with Your Shadow.* Minneapolis, MN: Augsburg Publishing.

*Minuchin, S. (1977) *Families and Family Therapy.* London: Tavistock.

Moore, J. (1984) Caring for the carers. *Nursing Times* **80**(41): 28–30.

Moorey, S. & Greer, S. (1989) *Psychological Therapy for Patients with Cancer.* Oxford: Heinemann.

*Mucchielli, R. (1972) *Face to Face in the Counselling Interview.* London: Macmillan.

*Munro, A. et al. (1989) *Counselling: The Skills of Problem-Solving.* London: Routledge.

*Murgatroyd, S. (1985) *Counselling and Helping.* London: Methuen.

*Murgatroyd, S. et al. (1982) *Coping with Crisis.* Milton Keynes: Open University Press.

*Murgatroyd, S. et al. (1985) *Helping Families in Distress.* Milton Keynes: Open University Press.

Navone, J. (1977) *Towards a Theology of Story.* Slough: St Paul Publications.

*Nelson-Jones, R. (1982) *Theory and Practice of Counselling Psychology*. London: Cassell.

*Nelson-Jones, R. (1984) *Personal Responsibility Counselling and Therapy*. Milton Keynes: Open University Press.

Nelson-Jones, R. (1988) *Practical Counselling and Helping Skills* (2nd edn). London: Cassell.

Nisbet, R. (1969) In Egan, G. & Cowan, R.M. (1979) *People in Systems, an Integrative Approach to Human Development*. Belmont, CA: Brooks/Cole.

*Noonan, E. (1983) *Counselling Young People*. London: Methuen.

Nouwen, H.J., McNeill, D.P. & Morrison, D.A. (1982) *Compassion*. London: Darton, Longman & Todd.

Nurse, G. (1978) What is counselling? *Midwife, Health Visitor and Community Nurse* **14**(10): 352–355.

Nurse, G. (1980) *Counselling and the Nurse* (2nd edn). Aylesbury: HM & M.

*Ogier, M.E. (1989) *Working and Learning*. London: Scutari.

Ogier, M. & Cameron-Buccheri, R. (1990) Supervision: a cross-cultural approach. *Nursing Standard* **4**(31): 24–26.

Olson-Dorland, G. (1969) *A Reference Handbook and Dictionary of Nursing*. Philadelphia: W.B. Saunders.

Partridge, K.B. (1978) Nursing values in a changing society. *Nursing Outlook* **26**(6): 356–360.

*Patterson, C. (1986) *Theories of Counselling and Psychotherapy*. London: Harper & Row.

Pearson, A. (1983) *The Clinical Nursing Unit*. London: Heinemann.

Pembrey, S. (1987) Support your ward sister. *Nursing Times* **83**(39): 27–29.

Perls, F. (1973) *The Gestalt Approach and Eye Witness to Therapy*. New York: Bantam.

Perry, F. (1988) Far from black and white. *Nursing Times* **84**(10): 40–41.

Quilliam, S. & Grove-Stephenson, I. (1990) *The Counselling Handbook*. Wellingborough: Thorsons.

Raeburn, A. (1979) The nurses I know. *Nursing Times* **75**(32): 1346.

*Ram Dass & Gorman P. (1985) *How Can I Help?* London: Rider.

Riley, V.A. (1983) Counselling the mentally handicapped. *Counselling* **43**: 10–13.

Roach, M.S. (1985) Caring as responsivity: a response to value as the important-in-itself. Paper delivered at the 2nd International Congress on Nursing Law and Ethics, Tel Aviv.

Roach, M.S. (1987) *The Human Act of Caring: A Blueprint for the Health Professions*. Ottawa: Canadian Hospital Association.

*Roet, B. (1989) *A Safer Place to Cry*. London: Optima.

Rogers, C.R. (1942) *Counselling and Psychotherapy*. Boston: Houghton Mifflin.

Rogers, C.R. (1951) *Client-Centred Therapy*. Boston: Houghton Mifflin.

Rogers, C.R. (1957) In Scott, C. (1984) Empathy: examination of a crucial concept. *Counselling* **49**: 3–6.

Rogers, C.R. (1959) In Koch, S. (ed.) (1959) *Psychology: a Study of a Science*. New York: McGraw-Hill.

Rogers, C.R. (1961) *On Becoming a Person*. London: Constable.

Rogers, C.R. (1967) *The Therapeutic Relationship and its Impact*. Madison: University of Wisconsin.

Rogers, C.R. (1975) Empathic: an unappreciated way of being. *Counselling Psychologist* **21**: 95–103.

Rogers, C.R. (1978) *On Personal Power*. London: Constable.

Rogers, C.R. (1980) *A Way of Being*. Boston: Houghton Mifflin.

Salvage, J. (1990) The theory and practice of the 'new nursing'. *Nursing Times* occasional paper **86**(1): 42–45.

*Satir, V. (1978) *Peoplemaking*. London: Souvenir.

Scrutton, S. (1989) *Counselling Older People*. London: Edward Arnold.

Scully, R. (1981) Staff support groups: helping nurses to help themselves. *Journal of Nursing Administration* **11**(3): 48–51.

Sigman, P. (1979) Ethical choice in nursing. *Advances in Nursing Science* **1**(3): 37–52.

Simonton, S., Simonton, O.C. & Creighton, J.C. (1978) *Getting Well Again*. New York: Bantam.

*Smith, C. (1982) *Social Work with the Dying and Bereaved*. London: Macmillan.

Smith, P. (1989) Nurses' emotional labour. *Nursing Times* **85**(47):49–51.

Speck, P. (1978) *Loss and Grief in Medicine*. London: Baillière Tindall.

*Stewart, W. (1983) *Counselling in Nursing*. London: Harper & Row.

*Stewart, W. (1985) *Counselling in Rehabilitation*. London: Croom Helm.

Swaffield, L. (1988) Sharing the load. *Nursing Times* **84**(36): 24, 26.

Taylor, J.V. (1972) *The Go-Between God.* London: SCM Press.

Thiroux, J. (1980) *Ethics: Theory and Practice* (2nd edn). Encino, CA: Glencoe Publishing.

*Thompson, S. (1988) *Group Process and Family Therapy.* Oxford: Pergamon.

Tomlinson, A. (1983) *Communication Skills: Questioning.* Private circulation.

Townsend, I. & Linsley, W. (1980) Creating a climate for carers. *Nursing Times* **76**(27): 1180–1190.

Truax, C.B. (1961) A scale for the measurement of accurate empathy. *Psychiatric Institute Bulletin*, University of Wisconsin **1**, 12.

Tschudin, V. (1981) A question of mind over matter? *Nursing Times* **77**(10): 424–426.

Tschudin, V. (1989a) Ethics, morality and nursing. In Hinchliff, S.M., Norman, S.E. & Schober, J.E. (eds) (1989) *Nursing Practice and Health Care.* London: Edward Arnold.

Tschudin, V. (1989b) *Beginning with Empathy.* A facilitator's guide. Edinburgh: Churchill Livingstone.

Tschudin, V. (1989c) *Beginning with Empathy.* A learner's handbook. Edinburgh: Churchill Livingstone.

United Kingdom Central Council (1984) *Code of Professional Conduct for the Nurse, Midwife and Health Visitor.*

Walker, P. (1976) Taped interview. Private circulation.

Walsh, P. (1985) Speaking up for the patient. *Nursing Times* **81**(18): 24–27.

Wells, R. (1988) AIDS-related tumours. In Tschudin, V. (ed.) (1988) *Nursing the Patient with Cancer.* Hemel Hempstead: Prentice Hall.

Woolfe, R. (1989) *Counselling skills.* A Training Manual. Edinburgh: Scottish Health Education Group.

*Worden, J. (1983) *Grief Counselling and Grief Therapy.* London: Tavistock.

*Wright, R. (1986) *Caring in Crisis.* Edinburgh: Churchill Livingstone.

Index